Taoist Foreplay

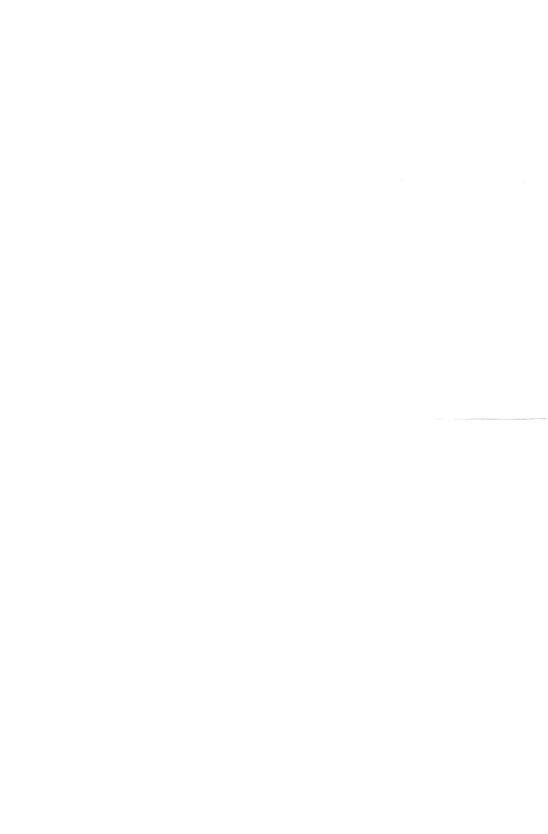

Taoist Foreplay

Love Meridians
and Pressure Points

Mantak Chia and Kris Deva North

Destiny Books
Rochester, Vermont • Toronto, Canada

Destiny Books
One Park Street
Rochester, Vermont 05767
www.DestinyBooks.com

Destiny Books is a division of Inner Traditions International

Library of Congress Cataloging-in-Publication Data
Chia, Mantak, 1944–
   Taoist foreplay : love meridians and pressure points / Mantak Chia and Kris Deva North.
       p. cm.
   "Originally published in Thailand in 2005 by Universal Tao Publications under the title A Touch of Sex."
   Includes bibliographical references and index.
   ISBN 978-1-59477-188-0 (pbk.)
 1. Sex instruction. 2. Sex—Religious aspects—Taoism. 3. Foreplay. 4. Acupressure. I. North, Kris Deva. II. Title.
   HQ56.C544 2010
   613.6'9—dc22

                                                            2010004012

Printed and bound in India by Replika Press Pvt. Ltd.

10   9   8   7   6   5   4   3

Photography by Michael Cullingworth, Ian Jackson, Red James, Kris Deva North, Sutharshini
Artwork by Ian Jackson, Beata Kociatyn, Jaclyn Snyders, Sutharshini
Research by Jaclyn Snyders
Thanks to Sue Hix for use of her meridian diagrams

Text design and layout by Virginia Scott Bowman
This book was typeset in Janson and Futura with Present and Diotima as display typefaces

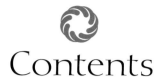

Contents

Acknowledgments   vii

Putting Taoist Foreplay into Practice   ix

1   Love, Sex, and Touch   1

2   Rivers of Love, Pools of Desire   10

3   Whole Body Love-Shiatsu   55

4   Self-Shiatsu: Care and Maintenance   112

5   Compatibility: Marriages Made in Heaven   131

Resources   152

Bibliography   154

About the Authors   156

The Universal Tao System   159

Index   160

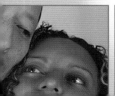
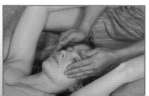
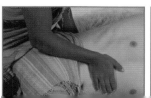
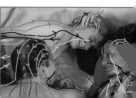

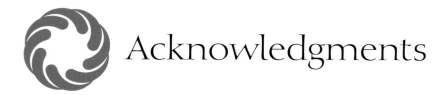# Acknowledgments

The Universal Tao Publications staff involved in the preparation and production of *Taoist Foreplay* extend our gratitude to the many generations of Taoist masters who have passed on their special lineage, in the form of an unbroken oral transmission, over thousands of years. We thank Taoist Master Yi Eng for his openness in transmitting the formulas of Taoist Inner Alchemy. We also wish to thank the thousands of unknown men and women of the Chinese healing arts who developed many of the methods and ideas presented in this book.

We offer our eternal gratitude to our parents and teachers for their many gifts to us. Remembering them brings joy and satisfaction to our continued efforts in presenting the Universal Tao System. For their gifts, we offer our eternal gratitude and love. As always, their contribution has been crucial in presenting the concepts and techniques of the Universal Tao.

We thank the many contributors essential to this book's final form: the editorial and production staff at Inner Traditions/Destiny Books for their efforts to clarify the text and produce a handsome new edition of the book.

We wish to thank the following people for their assistance in producing the original edition of this book: Michael Cullingworth, Ian Jackson, Red James, Beata Kociatyn, Jaclyn Snyders, Kris Deva North, and Sutharshini for photography and artwork; Sue Hix for authorizing the use of illustrations from her excellent classical meridian charts; Matt Lewis and anonymous others for donating their bodies to photography; Liz Peart and Ursula Gavin for their advice and support; Jaclyn Snyders for impeccable research, artwork, and tireless application.

Special thanks to teachers and students of the Zen School of Shiatsu in London who conscientiously investigated modern applications of ancient secrets and donated their time and talents to the creation of the ideas and illustrations. Finally, love and gratitude to Lee Dubens, Kris Deva North's cofounder of the Zen School, without whom none of this would have happened.

A special thanks goes to our Thai production team: Raruen Keawapadung, computer graphics, and Saniem Chaisarn, production designer.

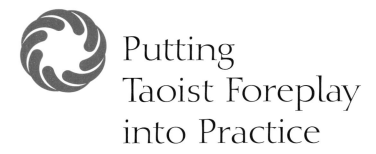

Putting Taoist Foreplay into Practice

The practices described in this book have been used successfully for thousands of years by Taoists trained by personal instruction. Readers should not undertake the practice without receiving personal transmission and training from a certified instructor of the Universal Tao, since certain of these practices, if done improperly, may cause injury or result in health problems. This book is intended to supplement individual training by the Universal Tao and to serve as a reference guide for these practices. Anyone who undertakes these practices on the basis of this book alone does so entirely at his or her own risk.

The meditations, practices, and techniques described herein are not intended to be used as an alternative or substitute for professional medical treatment and care. Any reader suffering from illnesses based on psychological or emotional disorders should consult an appropriate professional health care practitioner or therapist. Such problems should be corrected before you start training.

This book does not attempt to give any medical diagnosis, treatment, prescription, or remedial recommendation in relation to any human disease, ailment, suffering, or physical condition whatsoever.

The Universal Tao cannot be responsible for the consequences of any practice or misuse of the information in this book. If the reader undertakes any exercise without strictly following the instructions, notes, and warnings, the responsibility must lie solely with the reader.

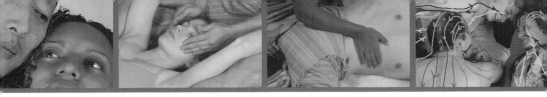

Love, Sex, and Touch

Your body is a landscape
of hills and valleys,
woodland glades,
caves of delight
pastures of pleasure,
stirred by breezes of bliss,
fed by rivers of desire,
watered by clouds and rain of ecstasy.

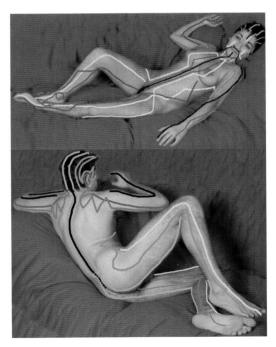

Fig. 1.1. The body is a landscape.

Nature has gifted us
with eyes to see these wonders,
ears to hear the sounds of love,
noses to smell the fragrance of passion,
tongues to taste the fruits of desire,
lips to kiss,
and hands to touch.

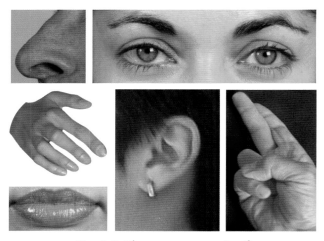

Fig. 1.2. The senses: nature's gift

Whoever you are—woman or man, straight, gay, or bi—you can become a far more effective lover! The act itself is natural. You know what to do. It is the moments leading up to the act that make it more or less pleasurable for you and your partner. As with cooking a Chinese meal, preparation is the key. Knowing the psycho-sensual secrets of certain pressure points and energy channels of the body will help you become a better lover, however good you are already (figs. 1.3 and 1.4). You may have discovered this for yourself, quite by chance. Using these secrets will help you to create and enjoy longer and more pleasurable sexual encounters. You will be able to prolong peak moments beyond bliss into ecstasy.

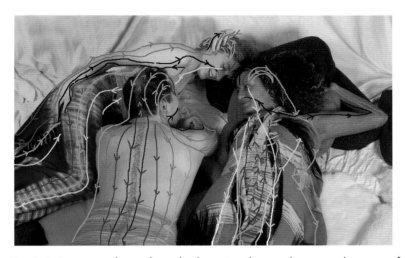

Fig. 1.3. Become a better lover by knowing the psycho-sensual secrets of pressure points and energy channels.

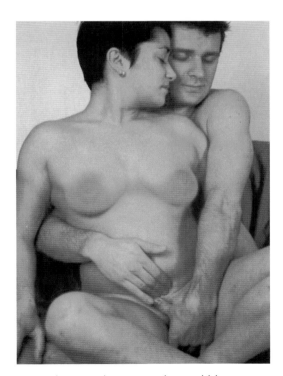

Fig. 1.4. Prolong peak moments beyond bliss into ecstasy.

THE ORIGINS AND HISTORY
OF TAOIST SEXUAL PRACTICES

When lovers first touched they invented what we call Love-Shiatsu. *Shiatsu* is a Japanese word meaning "finger-push." Sexual practices have been studied for centuries in both East and West. Chinese and Japanese traditions combined the study of sex with medicine based upon stimulation of certain pressure points. The Yellow Emperor, Huang Ti (2697–2598 BCE), codified the theory behind the therapy (fig. 1.5). Treatment, he decreed, should vary according to application, whether to heal or to stimulate and sustain sexual desire.

In its beginnings, Chinese medicine was clearly a departure from the practices of ancient shamans, who believed that illnesses were caused by bad spirits. The approach of the Yellow Emperor, on the

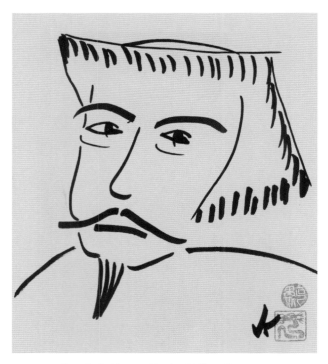

Fig. 1.5. Huang Ti, the Yellow Emperor

other hand, linked disease with factors such as diet, lifestyle, age, and environment. His approach was conveyed in the talks that he had with his personal physicians, recorded in the *Neijing*, the *Classic of Internal Medicine*. Health and disease were also understood in terms of forces and principles in the universe, particularly yin and yang, the five elements, and chi (life-force energy).

Yin and Yang

The concept of yin and yang is based on the dualistic principle of order that brings together contradictory principles and conditions. Yin and yang can stand for night and day, moon and sun, earth and sky, dark and light, cold and warm, matter and energy, or stillness and activity. Neither yin nor yang is considered to be "bad" or "good"; they are equally valued aspects of one unity. In Chinese medicine, being healthy means that yin and yang are in equilibrium. Illness results when the balance falls more to the side of either yin or yang.

The Five Elements

The five elements refer to five basic energy transformations that flow from the interactions of yin and yang. The physical elements found in nature (wood, fire, earth, metal, and water) are seen as symbolic expressions of the five tendencies of energy in motion. Wood represents energy that is developing and generating. Fire represents energy that is expanding and radiating. Earth represents energy that is stabilizing and centering. Metal represents energy that is solidifying and contracting. Water is energy that is conserving, gathering, and sinking. The five energies that give birth to the universe also form the organs and the personality. Thus, each human being, as a microcosm of these elemental energies, reflects the universe and its interacting forces. The model of the five elements provides helpful insights into the effect of mood on loving and indeed all aspects of relationship.

Chi: Life-force Energy

Traditional Chinese medicine sees chi as circulating through the human body through a series of channels or meridians. Lined up along the meridians like pearls on a string are the acupuncture or acupressure points. It is at these points that the meridians are connected to the surface of the body; by touching these points from the outside, energy can be moved. The pressure points of shiatsu are the same as the points used for acupuncture.

Oriental love-medicine takes a holistic view, in which meridians, organs, senses, emotions—the physical, energetic, and spiritual aspects of humanity—all interact.

Immortality and Sexuality

In the days of the Yellow Emperor they searched for immortality as the logical extension of perfect health. He is said to have attained it by having sex with 1,200 wives and concubines. The Queen Mother of the West likewise but with numbers unrecorded.

The emperor and his female advisor Su Nu are credited with creating the *Su Nu Ching*, a dialogue of sexual practice, which included exchanges such as the following:

Huang Ti: "And what is the method of nine shallow and one deep?"

Su Nu: "That means to thrust nine times shallow and then one deep, in time with the breath. Too shallow may not yield the greatest pleasure, too deep may be injurious."

Taoist practice has always been sexy. Four thousand years ago the top shelf was peopled with stories of the Yellow Emperor and the Queen Mother of the West. Nowadays we like one-to-one relationships and are perhaps skeptical of immortality. But we can enjoy the secrets that kept the Yellow Emperor going and the Queen Mother coming.

Sex Is the Servant, Not the Master

Taoists say that if the products of our pleasure are not being deployed to start new life, then we can internalize the intense energy, hormones, and nutrients to improve our own lives. From foreplay to climax, a Taoist controls and harvests the abundance of reproductive power otherwise wasted in unmindful intercourse.

Yang has the power to repopulate a continent in a single ejaculation, yin has eggs to generate hundreds of lives. The Taoist masters taught the emperors and their wives and concubines to recycle this potent life force and harmonize their cycles of pleasure through a process known as Inner Alchemy. Later Taoist sex manuals continued the tradition of treating both genders as equal, but as dynasties came and went, mixed fortunes followed for the practices.

Sex and the Dynasties

The Chou Dynasty (770 BCE to 222 BCE) had a Taoist doctrine although Taoism was not yet a formal religion. Women were thought to have an inexhaustible supply of yin essence. A man who ejaculated or used up his yang essence without absorbing enough yin could experience health problems and even death.

The Ch'in Dynasty (221 BCE to 24 CE) changed from Taoism to the quite different Confucianism, which considered women inferior. Sex was considered to be for procreation only, otherwise sinful. However, religious and magical Taoism peacefully coexisted with behavioral Confucianism.

A Taoist resurgence in the Later Han Dynasty (25 CE to 220 CE) saw the rehabilitation of sexual practices and the reappearance of texts attributed to the Yellow Emperor. In the confusion of Three Kingdoms and Six Dynasties (221 CE to 590 CE) conflicts arose between Taoist, Confucian, and the newly arriving Buddhist doctrines. The rise of Buddhism under the Northern Wei (386 to 534 CE) led to persecution of practitioners of the old ways. Healing and sexual practices became politicized.

Then in the Sui Dynasty (590 CE to 618 CE) Taoism again became the official religion and sexual literature flourished. *Secret Instructions of the Jade Bedchamber* appeared. It is a Taoist text on harmonizing male (yang) and female (yin) energies for mutual nourishment—yin drawing on yang and yang from yin. It declares that single, dual, and multiple energy cultivation can be practiced for pleasure, health, longevity, healing, self-realization, and, ultimately, experiencing a self beyond the cycle of life and death.

Under the Tang Dynasty (618 CE to 960 CE) Taoism became "the Establishment." Physicians in the Tang Dynasty, who vivisected condemned prisoners, described flows of energy through invisible channels, which excited certain sensations in different parts of the body, ceasing at the moment of death. They speculated that if this flow could be sustained . . . it might offer healing and even immortality.

From later Sung to the present, various forms of Taoism evolved, in which some Buddhist and Confucian doctrines were integrated. Chinese alchemists sought an elixir to render their emperors immortal and perpetually potent. This external alchemy lost its appeal when it dispatched a few courtiers and kings as well as a number of alchemists. But the search for eternal health and infinite pleasure continued.

While the *Neijing*, the *Classic of Internal Medicine*, became the source for most Chinese medical literature, the classics on the "Art of the Bedchamber" are still widely quoted in almost every Oriental sex publication in both East and West. The shiatsu pressure points for infinite pleasure indefinitely prolonged were passed down through the secret lineages of the Fang Shi.

RUNNING WATER DOES NOT STAGNATE

Nowadays we are not emperors and empresses. We go to work, we play, we sleep. Our society has different problems to cope with. Rather than having our heads cut off for speaking out of turn we are more likely to experience stress in the workplace, leading to heart problems and other such diseases. But we still ingest toxic substances for moments of immortality. And we still have sex. Our modern-day ideal is to have a nice meal, a bottle of wine, and frantic sex. If everything goes as we hope, we will climax at the same time. Then we'll fall asleep or go take a shower.

We can benefit from the ancient perspective that regarded sex as healthy, fun, and serious business: If you want to understand the business of life, then you need to examine the business of where life starts and where life ends . . . the business of the bedchamber.

The ancient teachings also help us to understand the differences between men and women and how harmonizing these differences results in better loving. Women fear insensitivity. Men fear inability to perform. Both fear rejection. Are you aroused more quickly, your partner more slowly? It is quite usual for the man to climax first. Woman comes to the boil more slowly but simmers longer. He's done in, she's ready for more.

Shiatsu secrets help modern lovers harmonize different cycles of arousal:

- For longer and more pleasurable sexual encounters
- To sustain the intensity of first love through all the seasons of maturing relationship
- To avoid energy loss
- To maintain good sexual health: running water does not stagnate

These secrets are based on intimate knowledge of the flow of energy.

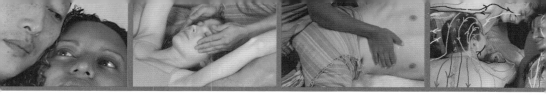

Rivers of Love,
Pools of Desire

The sexual and healing practices developed in the rural communities of ancient China still work today because they make sense. The ancients noticed that just as rivers flow through the countryside, irrigating fields and accumulating in pools or watering holes, energy flows between the organs of the body along meridians and accumulates in points. In a modern city the meridians are the streets, the points are the intersections, junctions, and places of access, and the organs are the locations around them.

In the countryside the weather affects the landscape, resulting sometimes in flooding, sometimes in drought, and often in effective irrigation. In the city circulation undergoes peak times and slack times, and sometimes things break down. Similarly, our energy sometimes circulates smoothly, but is also subject at times to blocks and imbalances, which affect our well-being and moods.

THE FIVE PHASES
OF ENERGY

The Chinese laws of support and control offer deep insights into the relationships among the five phases of energy that operate at all levels from the microcosmic to the macrocosmic. These energies are represented in multiple interlocking cycles including: 1) five seasons of the year—spring, summer, Indian summer, fall, and winter; 2) five phases of creation—becoming, growing, ripening, harvesting, and perishing (or becoming dormant); 3) five natural elements—wood, fire, earth, metal, and water; and 4) five pairs of internal organs in the body—liver/gallbladder, heart/small intestine, spleen/stomach, lungs/large intestine, and kidneys/bladder. Each element also has positive and negative emotions associated with it. Thus the liver, for example, is linked to the element wood, the season spring, the sprouting of new growth, desire, and anger, and the heart is associated with the element fire, the season summer, the time of blossoming, passion, and impatience (see fig. 2.1 on page 12).

TAOIST RELATIONSHIPS
BETWEEN HUMANS AND NATURAL CYCLES

QUALITY				
Elements	Wood	Fire	Earth	Metal	Water
Phases of creation	Becoming	Blossoming	Ripening	Harvesting	Perishing (dormancy)
Seasons	Spring	Summer	Indian Summer	Fall	Winter
Human organs	Liver/ Gallbladder	Heart/ Small intestine	Spleen (and Pancreas)/ Stomach	Lungs/ Large intestine	Kidneys/ Bladder
Emotions	Desire/ Anger	Passion/ Impatience	Calm/ Worry	Boldness/ Misery	Gentleness/ Fear

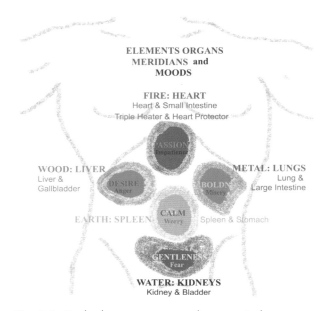

Fig. 2.1. Each element corresponds to particular organs,
meridians, and emotions.

ELEMENTS AND MERIDIANS

Each element is associated with organ-meridian networks that are designated as either yin or yang. Yin and yang are generally used to describe the relationships between things. For example, men are more yang and women more yin, but among both men and women are those more yin or yang in comparison with others of the same gender. Fire is more yang, water more yin, but a candle is more yin than the sun and a wave more yang than a tear drop. Harmonizing extremes of yin and yang can enhance relationships, whether with a lover or between aspects of your self.

Yin meridians relate to inner aspects of the body and correspond with the deeper organs: heart, lungs, liver, spleen, and kidney. The yang channels relate to the outer aspects and network the more hollow organs: the intestines, bladder, and gallbladder. The yin meridians can be thought of as relating to the more inner, emotional, and spiritual aspects and the yang to the more physical and mundane.

To picture the meridians, think of a person with arms extended upward.

- The yin meridians run along the front of the body from bottom to top (from the ground to the body to the sky).
- The yang meridians—with one exception—run along the back of the body from top to bottom (from sky to the body to the earth).
- A yin meridian is always paired with a yang meridian. In this way traditional Chinese medicine sees each person as part of the energy circulation between the sky (yang) and the earth (yin).
- The meridians are named after the internal organs as they are described in traditional Chinese medicine.

THE FIVE ELEMENTS AND OUR EMOTIONS

Different aspects of organ-meridian networks exert influences on one another, some nourishing, some regulating (see fig. 2.2 on page 14). Their nourishing influences are expressed as the "Cycle of Support," and their regulating influences are expressed as "Lines of Control."

CYCLE OF SUPPORT
Wood feeds fire
Fire feeds earth
Earth feeds metal
Metal feeds water
Water feeds wood
LINES OF CONTROL
Wood regulates earth
Earth regulates water
Water regulates fire
Fire regulates metal
Metal regulates wood

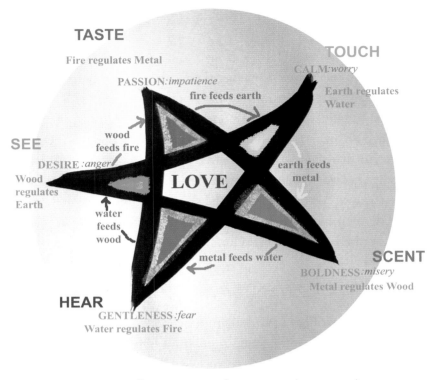

TASTE

Fire regulates Metal

PASSION:*impatience*

fire feeds earth

TOUCH

CALM:*worry*

Earth regulates Water

SEE

wood feeds fire

DESIRE :*anger*

Wood regulates Earth

LOVE

earth feeds metal

water feeds wood

metal feeds water

SCENT

BOLDNESS:*misery*

Metal regulates Wood

HEAR

GENTLENESS:*fear*

Water regulates Fire

Fig. 2.2. Different aspects of organ-meridian networks
exert influences on one another, some nourishing
(Cycle of Support), some regulating (Lines of Control).

Moods, health, and well-being are ruled by the interplay between the five elements. Knowledge of the elements can aid you in soothing and regulating negative emotions and heightening positive ones

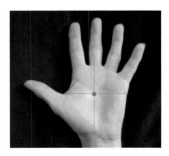

Fig. 2.3. Sense your lover's energy and mood with your palm.

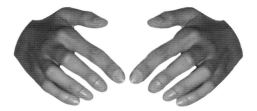

Fig. 2.4. Use your hands to calm things down or get things going.

in yourself and your lover. For example, seeing can lead to desire but if you don't get what you want, you may become impatient. You may find you can deal with your impatience with boldness or, on the other hand, fear (usually fear of rejection) may control your impatience.

You can use the diagrams (figs. 2.1 and 2.2) to work out how moods can affect one another. This will help you to see how you can affect your moods: drawing on their energy rather than being drained by them. Knowledge of elements and meridians helps you choose appropriate responses to the moods of your lover, making for better loving, both outside and inside the bedroom. Sensations of heat or coolness tell the story of elemental imbalances. You can use your palm to scan the energy or touch the flesh of your partner to sense your lover's mood (fig. 2.3). Then you can use your hands to calm things down or get things going (fig. 2.4).

THE FIRE ELEMENT

Fire dances, fire warms, fire burns, fire creates, and fire destroys.

The sun shines, fire nourishing earth, nourished by wood, controlling metal, controlled by water.

Passion is the virtue of fire energy in its positive aspect, while the negative emotion is impatience.

The sense of the fire element is the sense of taste, and the feature is the tongue. What is the taste of your lover?

The color of fire is red, its season is summer, direction is south, and the guardian animal is the Firebird (see fig. 2.5 on page 16).

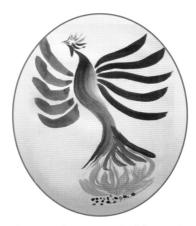

Fig. 2.5. The guardian animal of fire is the Firebird.

Fire Element Meridians

There are four meridians of the fire element: Heart, Small Intestine, Triple Heater, and Heart Protector (or Pericardium).

Heart: Yin Meridian

Heart is the sovereign organ, ruler of body/mind/spirit: a position of great responsibility. Approach the Heart meridian with respect, using the services of the other fire channels to come close to the monarch. The Heart channel flows through nine points along the edge of the inner arm, from the armpit to the tip of the little finger (figs. 2.6 and 2.7).

Although the sensory organ of the Heart meridian is the tongue, the spirit of the heart shines in the eyes. Can you read your lover's heart in your lover's eyes?

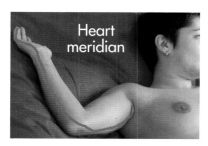

Fig. 2.6. Heart: yin meridian

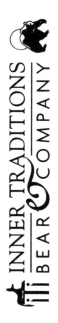

INNER TRADITIONS
BEAR & COMPANY

Inner Traditions • Bear & Company
P.O. Box 388
Rochester, VT 05767-0388
U.S.A.

PLEASE SEND US THIS CARD TO RECEIVE OUR LATEST CATALOG.

Book in which this card was found _____

❑ Check here if you would like to receive our catalog via e-mail.

Name_____ Company_____

Address_____ Phone_____

City_____ State_____ Zip_____ Country_____

E-mail address_____

Please check the following area(s) of interest to you:

❑ Health   ❑ Self-help   ❑ Science/Nature   ❑ Shamanism

❑ Ancient Mysteries ❑ New Age/Spirituality   ❑ Ethnobotany   ❑ Martial Arts

❑ Spanish Language ❑ Sexuality/Tantra   ❑ Children   ❑ Teen

Please send a catalog to my friend:

Name_____ Company_____

Address_____ Phone_____

City_____ State_____ Zip_____ Country_____

Order at 1-800-246-8648 • Fax (802) 767-3726

E-mail: customerservice@InnerTraditions.com • Web site: www.InnerTraditions.com

Entering the presence of heart, or the beloved who rules your heart, sink to one knee in the traditional posture of proposal (fig. 2.8).

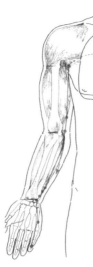

Fig. 2.7. The channel of the Heart flows along the edge of the inner arm, from the armpit to the tip of the little finger.

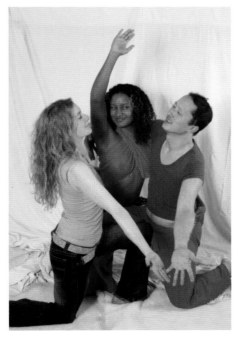

Fig. 2.8. Heart is passion, love, and joy; extending your arms and hands in an open embrace or reaching upward is the way to exercise the Heart meridian flowing along the inner arm.

Small Intestine: Yang Meridian

A little further from the center of the imperial court of the heart, the Small Intestine meridian is a more playful prospect altogether. Somewhat unruly and with a passion for life, this organ-meridian network twists and turns and dances (fig. 2.9).

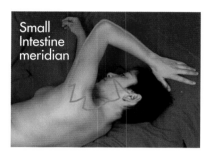

Fig. 2.9. Small Intestine: yang meridian

The Small Intestine meridian takes the fire energy of the heart through nineteen points from the outer edge of the pinkie up the outer edge of the hand and arm, zigzagging across the shoulder blade, up the side of the neck, across the cheek and back, to just in front of the ear (fig. 2.10).

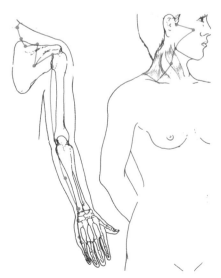

Fig. 2.10. The fire energy goes up the outer edge of the arm, through the shoulder blade and up to just in front of the ear.

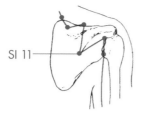

Fig. 2.11. Location of SI 11

Ease the shoulders with gentle palm or focused finger at SI 11 (fig. 2.11).

This meridian also indicates the ability to choose, as in the process of the organ itself, which takes the nutrients it needs from food in the digestive process and lets the waste pass through.

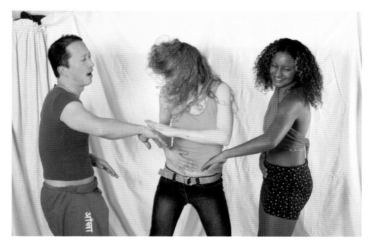

Fig. 2.12. Just as the Small Intestine meridian twists and turns and dances, dancing with twists and turns can give it a good workout.

Triple Heater: Yang Meridian

Triple Heater means "three cooking pots," representing the three levels of temperature in our being: hot around the head and heart where the fire energy flares, warm around the belly, the home of earth energy, and cool around the kidneys and bladder, source of our water energy. It runs through twenty-three points from the tip of the fourth or ring finger up the back of the hand and back of the arm, along the back of the shoulder, then up to the neck, behind and around the ear and past the temple to the outer end of the eyebrow (figs. 2.13 and 2.14).

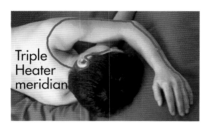

Fig. 2.13. Triple Heater: yang meridian

This prosaically mystical meridian has—like the lotus—its head in fire or facing the sun, its roots in water, and, unlike other meridians, has no particular organ association, though it could be connected with the diaphragms that unite the upper and lower sections of the torso.

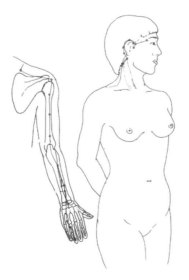

Fig. 2.14. The Triple Heater meridian runs from the tip of the fourth or ring finger to the outer end of the eyebrow.

The Triple Heater point (TH 1) on the fourth finger (fig. 2.15) is very good for soothing irritability: a gentle squeeze, perhaps, or a kiss? Some might say the best use for TH 1 is for putting on a ring.

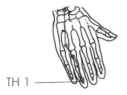

TH 1

Fig. 2.15. Location of TH 1

The Triple Heater distributes love energy around the meridian network, carrying the spark of life from its partner, Heart Protector, and circulating it through the source points. By applying your love energy to your lover's Triple Heater you affect all the dimensions of his or her energy body (fig. 2.16).

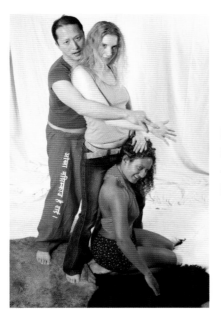

Fig. 2.16. Exercising the Triple Heater meridian is very easy: whenever you give someone a hug it gets a very nice stretch.

Heart Protector: Yin Meridian

Heart Protector, also known as Master of the Heart and Minister of Fun, carries the messages of the heart. This meridian comes to life at the time you are most likely to be setting out in search of fun: the cocktail hour, the time of the promenade.

The associated organ is the pericardium, a thick membrane around the heart itself. Heart Protector guards the way to the heart: spend time on this meridian to touch your lover's heart. If you are wearing your heart on your sleeve, it is likely to be on this meridian.

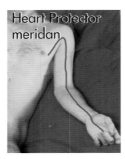

Fig. 2.17. Heart Protector: yin meridian

Starting between the ribs just two finger's width outside of the nipple, this meridian flows through nine points along the middle of the inside of the arm to the tip of the middle finger (fig. 2.17, 2.18, and 2.19). In energy terms, Heart Protector takes the first spark of life

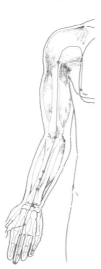

Fig. 2.18. Starting between the ribs just two finger's width outside of the nipple, this meridian flows along the middle of the inside of the arm to the tip of the middle finger.

crackling between the two kidneys and passes it to its partner, Triple Heater, for circulation around the organ-meridian networks.

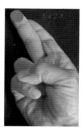

Fig. 2.19. Location of HP 1. HP 1 gets straight to the point. This is your favorite tool for focused penetration.

The HP 8 point, known as Labor's Love, is a true power point for both sending and receiving love energy (fig. 2.20). It can also be very calming, harmonizing imbalances of the spirit. Use it to soothe, to nurture, to arouse and excite passion. It is probably the point you will most use to connect with your lover. Place this point on any other and feel things start to stir. Leave it in place long enough and you will feel almost as if your energy fields are blending together.

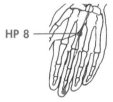

Fig. 2.20. Location of HP 8, Labor's Love, which is accessed through the palm of the hand

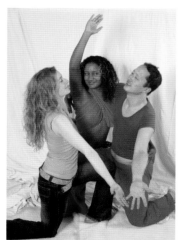

Fig. 2.21. Look out for opportunities to stretch the middle finger as well as the whole Heart Protector meridian.

THE EARTH ELEMENT

Earth is still. Earth is our Mother and provides all our needs. Everything we use comes from the earth and requires only work to transform it into anything from a spaceship to a wheelbarrow.

Deep in earth metal is born. Earth supports water, is held in place by wood, and nourished by fire, as the sun shines on the earth, giving light and life.

Calmness is the virtue of earth energy in its positive aspect, while the negative emotion is worry.

The sense of the earth element is the sense of touch, and the feature is the mouth. What more potent touch is there than a kiss? It is elaborated in all the sensual pleasure that leads to and from a kiss, until the ultimate kiss, and in all the pleasures of touch: stroking, caressing, and embracing.

The color of earth is yellow, and its season is harvest time when the fields are yellow and gold; the direction is the center and the guardian animal is the Golden Phoenix (fig. 2.22).

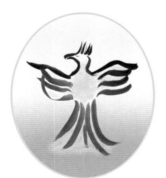

Fig. 2.22. The guardian animal of earth is the Golden Phoenix.

Earth Element Meridians

The meridians of the earth element are Stomach and Spleen.

Stomach: Yang Meridian

The Stomach meridian is the "yang in the yin"—it is the only yang meridian that crosses through the yin area of the front of the body.

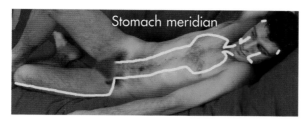

Fig. 2.23. Stomach: yang meridian

It runs vertically downward from the center of the lower edge of the eye socket to the edges of the mouth and past the outside of the jaws. One branch of the meridian returns upward past the ear to the temple. The main meridian continues along the lower jaw to the upper collarbone and from there straight down to the chest. It continues along the edge of the main abdominal muscles to the groin. From there it passes along the thigh and calf to the top of the foot; it ends on the outer edge of the nail of the second toe (figs. 2.23 and 2.24).

Stomach sees what it wants and goes for it. This is the meridian of survival, taking you forward to feast your eyes and fill your belly. Survival also refers to survival of the species, which relates to the stimulation and gratification of other senses.

If the way to a man's heart is through his stomach, the way to win a woman is to spend time on the Stomach meridian.

The point ST 17, known as the Breast Palace, is a strong feminine

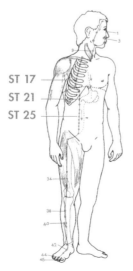

ST 17
ST 21
ST 25

Fig. 2.24. Starting with the eyes, the Stomach meridian flows down the length of the body, through the nipples, belly, and (in women) the ovarian tubes, along the outside of the front of the leg to the second and third toes.

arousal point, stimulating nipple/vulva connection while nurturing, soothing, and harmonizing heart and mind (fig. 2.25). It is also the starting point for the beautiful and sensual Massage of the Nine Flowers, given in Part Five of Love-Shiatsu (see chapter 3).

Two other important points of this meridian—ST 21 and ST 25—are on the route of the Nine Flowers, marching down to heaven at point CV 1, the beginning of the Conception Vessel (fig. 2.26). ST 21 is a very comforting point. ST 25, the Heavenly Axis, awakens sensuality and opens the belly to pleasure.

Caress down the line from tongue to toe with all the tools of your body; linger especially on ST 17.

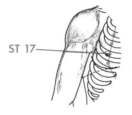

Fig. 2.25. ST 17, Breast Palace, is a strong feminine arousal point.

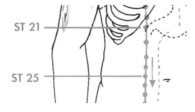

Fig. 2.26. ST 21 and ST 25, two points on the route of the Nine Flowers' path to heaven

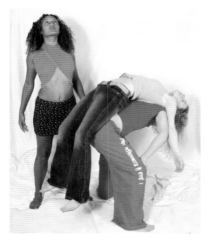

Fig. 2.27. Stretch the whole length of the body from head to toe. It helps to have a friend support you from below so you can just lean back and think of the Stomach meridian.

Spleen: Yin Meridian

The Spleen meridian lends itself to more intimate and sensual shiatsu, from sucking toes to stroking groin to caressing the outer edge of the breast (fig. 2.28). This meridian is for the subtle delights of the tease. The spleen also has the energy of nurturing and caring, following the nature of the earth element. Massaging along this meridian with love and care will bear fruit for your pleasure.

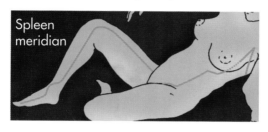

Fig. 2.28. Spleen: yin meridian

The Spleen meridian passes through twenty-one points starting from the big toe, running along the inside of the foot, past the inside of the ankle, and up to the inner calf and thigh to the groin region (fig. 2.29). From there, it runs sideways and then up to the upper abdomen, then along the chest, just beside the nipple. From there the

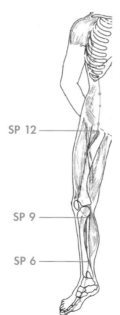

SP 12

SP 9

SP 6

Fig. 2.29. The Spleen meridian runs from the big toe to just beside the nipple.

meridian turns downward to run along the side of the body. The path of this meridian offers a journey of sensual delight.

There are three important Love-Shiatsu points along this meridian: SP 12, SP 9, and SP 6 (figs. 2.30, 2.31, and 2.32). Gently stroking or simply holding SP 12 with a still palm generates a feeling of warmth and pleasure across the genital area. SP 9 is a good point for men: it helps soothe pain in the genitals and controls wet dreams—keep your lover's juices just for you.

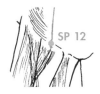

Fig. 2.30. Location of SP 12 in the groin

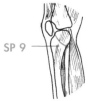

Fig. 2.31. Location of SP 9 near the knee

SP 6, Meeting of 3 Yin point, is a versatile point; it is helpful for conditions of impotence, frigidity, and premature ejaculation. Other uses include regulating menstruation, control of uterine bleeding, relieving pain of external genitals, treating sterility, seminal emissions, prolapse of the uterus, and difficult labor.

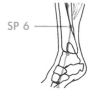

Fig. 2.32. Location of SP 6 above the ankle

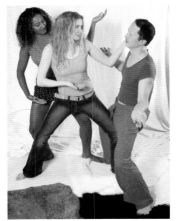

Fig. 2.33. The Spleen meridian likes movement to contrast with its duties of stillness: keeping things in place. Sometimes people need keeping in place, too.

THE METAL ELEMENT

Metal reflects and inspires, cuts and contains; it is the element of mystery, of swords and shields, coins, boxes, and silver-backed mirrors. Ancient alchemists sought to transform base metal into gold, a metaphor for transmutation of lust into love.

Born in the depths of earth, metal nourishes water. Its sharp edge controls wood and is itself controlled by fire as in the blacksmith's forge.

Metal's virtue is boldness and its negative emotion is misery, with associations of loneliness, isolation, sadness, and depression, especially the sadness of loss or unrequited love.

The sense of the metal element is smell, thus the nose is the feature of metal. The nose is sensitive to aphrodisiacs of fragrance, the scent of sex, evocative and provocative.

The color of metal is white, the direction is west, the season is autumn, and the guardian animal is the White Tiger (fig. 2.34).

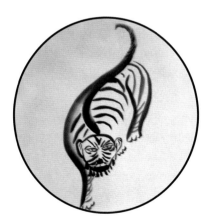

Fig. 2.34. The guardian animal of metal
is the White Tiger.

Metal Element Meridians

The meridians of metal are the Lung and the Large Intestine.

Lung: Yin Meridian

To breathe in is inspiration, to breathe out is to expire. The breath of life flows like a tide. The Lung meridian relates to our ability to take in life. It also governs the skin through which we breathe, and the hair on the body. Massage along the line of the Lung meridian to inspire the love of life in your beloved (fig. 2.35).

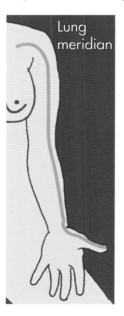

Fig. 2.35. Massage along the line of the Lung meridian to inspire the love of life in your beloved.

The Lung meridian is connected to the body surface at eleven points (fig. 2.36). It starts at the upper front of the rib cage, in the space between the top ribs, from where it goes slightly up and then across to the shoulder, down the inside of the upper arm, elbow, and lower arm, along the outside of the thumb to the thumbnail.

LU 1, Central Palace, is an important point along the Lung meridian (fig. 2.37). It is a beautiful place to rest your weight on your palms, soothing your lover's chest and ready to just slide down a little farther.

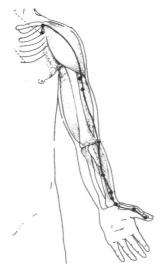

Fig. 2.36. The Lung meridian runs from the front of the shoulder along the edge of the inner arm to the thumb.

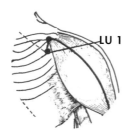

LU 1

Fig. 2.37. Location of LU 1 on the front of the shoulder

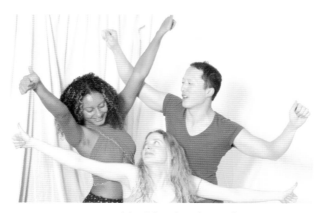

Fig. 2.38. Inspired by life! Thumbs up for exercise, breath, and vitality: a good way to stretch the Lung Meridian.

Large Intestine: Yang Meridian

The Large Intestine or Great Eliminator meridian has to do with getting rid of the waste from within. And why not from without? It's related season is autumn. Sometimes love has had its day, the season's over, and it's time to let go. As it is a meridian of the metal element, it is related to cutting, but it also works for containing.

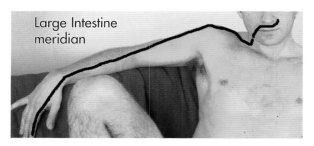

Fig. 2.39. Large Intestine: yang meridian

The Large Intestine meridian runs through twenty points from the nail of the index finger, on the side closest to the thumb, along the index finger across the hand and wrist, along the outside of the lower arm and elbow, and along the upper arm up to the shoulder (figs. 2.29 and 2.40). From there it runs sideways along the neck up to the corner of the mouth. Above the mouth it crosses over the upper lip to the opposite side, to end at the place where the corner of the nostril meets the face.

LI 4 is a great point for dealing with hangovers and visits to the dentist. It is good for encouraging elimination too (fig. 2.41). Press here when constipated, in pain, or both.

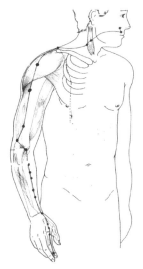

Fig. 2.40. The Large Intestine meridian runs from the tip of the forefinger along the edge of the outer arm to the place where the corner of the nostril meets the face.

LI 4

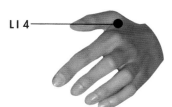

Fig. 2.41. Location of LI 4

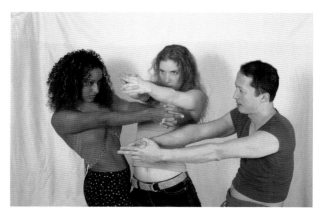

Fig. 2.42. Making or even stretching a point is a great exercise for the Large Intestine meridian. Or are they just encouraging elimination?

THE WATER ELEMENT

Crashing waves have been a sexual image since the invention of cinema.

Did life begin when lightning struck the ocean? If water holds the power of life, it can also carry the power of destruction. It was a flood that ended Noah's world.

Water is nature's shape-shifter, freezing solid as ice, boiling to steam, flowing as a teardrop or a tidal wave. As plain water it adapts to any shape, fits in any container, and, left to its own devices, always flows down to find the lowest level—a good thing to remember when "going with the flow."

Rivers flow into the ocean, which evaporates into clouds, which rain on the earth and refill the rivers. Water nourishes plant life, wood, and is nourished by the rocks of its sources, metal. Riverbanks and oceans are held in place by earth. And water controls fire, as you know from the barbecue and the fire brigade.

Water's virtue is gentleness and its emotion fear.

The sense of the water element is the sense of hearing: the ears are the features of water. "If music be the food of love . . ." and in relationship, how important it is to be heard by your lover.

Water's color is blue, its direction is north, and its season is winter, the time of death and conception. Water's guardian animal is the Black Tortoise or the Blue Tortoise (fig. 2.43).

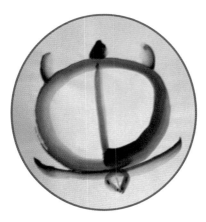

Fig. 2.43. One of the guardian animals of water is the Black Tortoise.

Water Element Meridians

Urinary Bladder and Kidney are the water meridians.

Urinary Bladder: Yang Meridian

The Urinary Bladder meridian runs behind us, the length of the back, connecting with the past (fig. 2.44). It routes through the ganglia, bunches of nerves along the spine related to the autonomic nervous system, which looks after both arousal and relaxation.

There is a strong energetic connection between the eye and arousal energy. From ancient Chinese and Japanese pillow books to the Internet porn of our present time, lovers have used visual imagery for sexual stimulation. The eye messages buzz along the nerves down to the sacrum, the triangular bone through which the Urinary Bladder meridian runs, and then shoot forward into the sexual area.

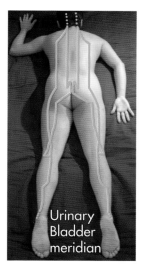

Fig. 2.44. Urinary Bladder: yang meridian

The Urinary Bladder meridian is the longest of the twelve main meridians. It runs through sixty-seven points, starting at the inner corner of the eye, from where it flows back over the head to the top of the spine (fig. 2.45). From here it divides into two branches, which run down the back almost parallel to each other. The inner branch continues downward past the sacrum and the inside of the buttock to the back of the thigh. The outer branch runs almost parallel across the middle of the buttock and along the back of the thigh to the knee. Here the inner and outer branches merge. Crossing the back of the calf and the outer edge of the foot, the meridian ends at the little toe.

By massaging the length of the Urinary Bladder meridian you can send a love-message through your partner's whole being.

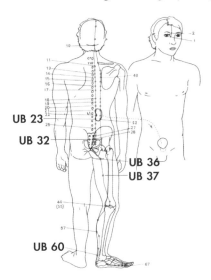

Fig. 2.45. The Urinary Bladder meridian starts at the inner corner of the eye, flows back over the head and down either side of the spine, down the back of the legs and along the edge of the foot to the little toe.

The Urinary Bladder meridian has five important points for Love-Shiatsu: UB 23, UB 32, UB 36, UB 37, UB 60.

UB 23 is the Kidney connector point. It supports sexual vitality for both sexes and enhances male stamina (fig. 2.46).

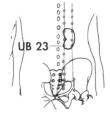

Fig. 2.46. Location of UB 23

UB 32 connects with the sacral nerves, which transmit arousal and arousal signals to the sexual area (fig. 2.47). Use the palm to hold this point for a long time.

A nice spiral massage at UB 36, the Supporting Palace, stimulates arousal in both sexes (fig. 2.48).

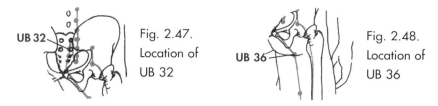

Fig. 2.47. Location of UB 32

Fig. 2.48. Location of UB 36

Touching UB 37 warms the whole leg and sends the love signals both ways (fig. 2.49).

Pinching UB 60, Kunlun Mountain, will give you a good idea of the strength of your partner's libido: the stiffer the stronger! This is also a useful point to press during labor (fig. 2.50).

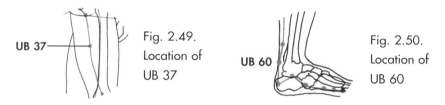

Fig. 2.49. Location of UB 37

Fig. 2.50. Location of UB 60

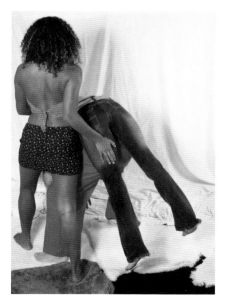

Fig. 2.51. Stretch the Bladder meridian by leaning forward or have your partner lift you. Just dangle, and feel the channel open.

Kidney: Yin Meridian

The Kidney meridian, guardian of ancestral chi and storehouse of genetic energy, holds the reproductive essence (fig. 2.52). The spark that is passed from generation to generation is the moving chi between the kidneys, captured by the Heart Protector and transmitted to the Triple Heater for circulation, constantly regenerating our life cycle in this life.

Kidney governs the bones, latticed crystalline structures sensitive to the transmission of etheric waves (the first radio sets used crystals). In shamanic traditions of many first nations, changing the bones is a step necessary for transformation.

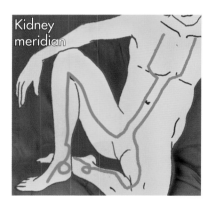

Fig. 2.52. Kidney: yin meridian

Connecting with the Kidney meridian is to connect with the essence of your lover's being. Touch this meridian and listen for the voices of the ancestors, and the descendants. Consisting of twenty-seven points, it begins on the sole of the foot about one-third of the way down from the toes, runs along the inner edge of the foot then up to circle the ankle; from there it continues up along the inside of the shin and thigh to the genitals, then up the chest to the collarbone (fig. 2.53).

There are three significant points to note along the Kidney meridian: KD 11, which relates to male sexual power, KD 3, or Great Stream, which can be used both for stimulation and balancing in both sexes, and KD 1, or Bubbling Spring, where you keep your feet on the ground (figs. 2.54, 2.55, and 2.56).

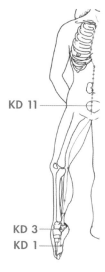

Fig. 2.53. The Kidney meridian starts in the sole of the foot, circles the ankle, and runs up the back of the inside leg, through the genitals, then up to the collarbone.

KD 11

KD 3

KD 1

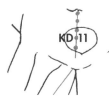

Fig. 2.54. Location of KD 11

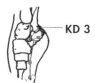

KD 3

Fig. 2.55. Location of KD 3, or Great Stream

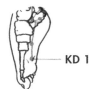

KD 1

Fig. 2.56. Location of KD 1, or Bubbling Spring, where you keep your feet on the ground

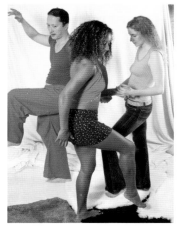

Fig. 2.57. Running water does not stagnate. Exercise the Kidney meridian with movement: stepping, stretching, and flowing.

THE WOOD ELEMENT

Spring is in the air! The wood element is the energy of birth, rebirth, and renewal, the unstoppability of life, the bursting of bud through bough.

Wood energy is dynamic, competitive (sometimes to the point of aggression), and powerful. Little plants grow in the brick walls of buildings and trees uproot the pavements of city streets.

Lust is in the air, in the springtime of life and in the springtime of a relationship.

Wood (tree, plant life) is the element of movement in all directions: roots penetrate down into the earth, the trunk rises erect toward heaven, and branches spread outward.

Trees compete for the light above and shade the earth below. Alive, they are nourished by water and their roots hold earth in place. They are cut by metal and provide fuel for fire.

Wood takes the conception energy of water and transforms it into lust for life: survival, sexual desire or continuation of the species, and the need to grow or progress.

Desire is the virtue of wood energy in its positive aspect, while the negative emotion is anger.

The sense of the wood element is the sense of sight, possibly our most powerful sense: 90 percent of our sensory input comes through

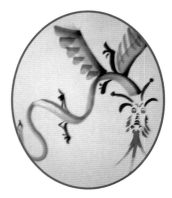

Fig. 2.58. The guardian animal of wood is the Dragon.

our eyes. Think of the depth of meaning in the words "We are seeing each other."

The color of wood is green, the direction is the east, where things begin, and the guardian animal is the Dragon (fig. 2.58).

Wood Element Meridians

The meridians of the wood element are Liver and Gall Bladder.

Liver: Yin Meridian

The Liver meridian is the channel of lust, desire in its most insistent and focused aspect. The meridian almost begs to be touched in all its length, from sucking the big toe to caressing along the inner thigh toward the Yin Gate or Jade Stalk (female and male organs of conception), and on up to just under the breast (fig. 2.59).

Liver is the energy of the element's season, springtime, of rising sap and urgent juices, the springtime of life itself, which will not be denied. Liver is competitive, the channel of natural selection, of fighting to win the prize of love. Competitive Liver energy extends into sport with its movement, focus, and desire to overcome.

The Liver meridian runs through fourteen points from the outer side of the big toe up the inside leg, through the pleasure zone of the inner thigh, right through the genital area and then up to just below the breast (see figs. 2.60 on page 42). To harness your lover's Liver

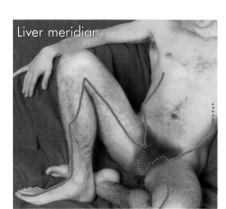

Liver meridian

Fig. 2.59. Liver: yin meridian

power, straddle the meridian, rubbing your CV 1 along its length and squeeze it with your PC (pubococcygeus) muscle along the way.

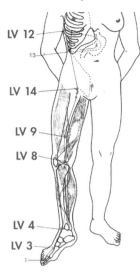

Fig. 2.60. The Liver meridian runs from the outer side of the big toe up the inside leg, through the pleasure zone of the inner thigh, right through the genital area to just below the breast.

There are six points of note along the Liver meridian: LV 14, LV 12, LV 9, LV 8, LV 4, LV 3.

LV 14, or Cyclic Gate, just below the underswell of the breast, is just waiting to be rubbed (fig. 2.61).

LV 12 is good for energy circulation and heightened sensitivity in the genital area (fig. 2.62).

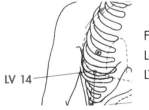

Fig. 2.61. Location of LV 14

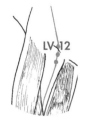

Fig. 2.62. Location of LV 12 in the groin

LV 9 is a subtle arousal point, situated on the pleasure muscles of the inner thigh approaching the sexual organs (fig. 2.63).

Regular massage of LV 8 improves sexual function (fig. 2.64).

Touching LV 4, Middle Barrier, is recommended to enhance male sexual energy (fig. 2.65).

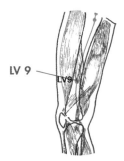

Fig. 2.63. Location of LV 9

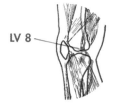

Fig. 2.64. Location of LV 8

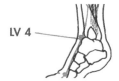

Fig. 2.65. Location of LV 4

LV 3, Great Rushing, is particularly recommended for enhancing female sexual energy (fig. 2.66).

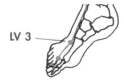

Fig. 2.66. Location of LV 3

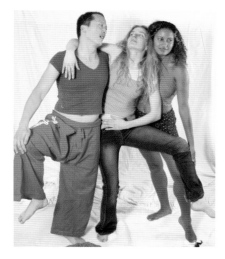

Fig. 2.67. Lift your knee in front then turn your leg out to the side for a good Liver meridian stretch. When lying down, simply open your legs to get a good stretch.

Gall Bladder: Yang Meridian

Gall Bladder looks after our lateral movement and is also known as the "Decision Maker." You can understand it by thinking about how you look from side to side as your mind goes "Will I? Won't I? Will I? Won't I?" The sides are special erogenous zones: when you feel your lover's hands slipping down the sides of your body to your hips in an early embrace, it's often a sign that some kind of spring is in the air (fig. 2.68).

The Gall Bladder meridian runs through fourteen points, starting at the outer edge of the eye then descending toward the ear (fig. 2.69). From there it rises to the temple and then drops down and circles the ear in a large arc. From the back of the ear it runs along the side of the skull in an arch back to the forehead. In another arch it runs back along the side of the head, down the neck, and along the shoulder muscles to the upper edge of the collarbone. From there it arcs around the front of the shoulder to the armpit and then in a zigzag down along the side of the body past the buttock and thigh. It then continues along the outside of the leg to run along the top of the foot to the base of the nail of the fourth toe.

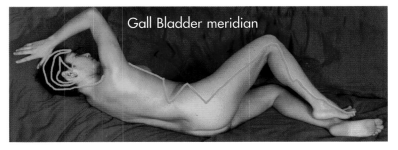

Fig. 2.68. Gall Bladder: yang meridian

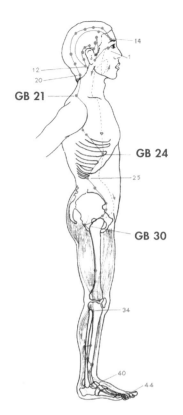

Fig. 2.69. The Gall Bladder meridian runs from the outer corner of the eyes all way down the sides of the body to the fourth toe.

There are three important points on the Gall Bladder meridian: GB 21, GB 24, GB 30.

GB 21, Shoulder Well, is one of the most effective points for relaxation and the beginnings of intimate contact (fig. 2.70). It also loosens a stiff neck and can help with difficult labor. As it is a powerful elimination point, it is unwise to use GB 21 in the early stages of pregnancy.

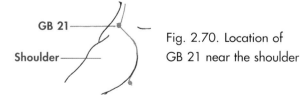

Fig. 2.70. Location of GB 21 near the shoulder

GB 24 warms the ribs and softens feelings of anxiety or indecision (fig. 2.71).

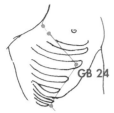

Fig. 2.71. Location of GB 24 toward the front of the ribs

GB 30, Jumping Circle, is a good starting point for a beautiful spiral massage around the buttocks (fig. 2.72).

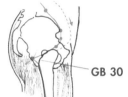

Fig. 2.72. Location of GB 30

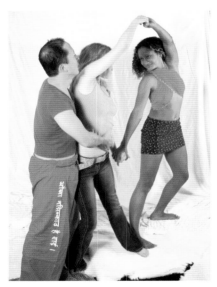

Fig. 2.73. Side stretches open the Gall Bladder meridian. Having a friend help with a pull makes for a stronger stretch.

GOVERNING VESSEL
AND CONCEPTION VESSEL MERIDIANS

The Governing and Conception Vessels do not form part of the organ-meridian networks of the five elements; they function instead to connect the elements of the earthly dimension with the powers of heaven and the universal life force or love energy. The Door of Life and the Gate of Life and Death are found on these two meridians.

Governing Vessel: Yang Meridian

With twenty-eight points, the Governing Vessel begins between the anus and the tip of the coccyx and runs up between the buttocks in a straight line along the spine and over the head toward the mouth. It ends at the upper lip (figs. 2.74 and 2.75).

The Governing Vessel connects the chakra energy centers of the back, from the sacrum—the sacred triangular bone at the base of the spine where the kundalini energy awaits arousal—to the Door of Life, a point between the second and third lumbar vertebrae. At the moment of conception, life from the universe enters our energy body through the Door of Life. From there it travels up through the back of the chakras, between the shoulder blades and up the back of the neck. There the spine, erect and hard, penetrates the soft moist warmth of the brain.

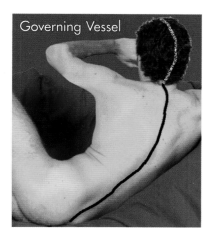

Fig. 2.74. Governing Vessel: yang meridian

This is the back channel of the Microcosmic Orbit, which links the chakras or energy centers and the belt channels, which spiral around them.

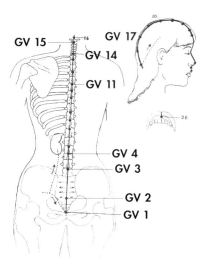

Fig. 2.75. Starting just above the anus, the route of the Governing Vessel runs up the back through the central nervous system, connecting the base of the body with the brain.

Several points along the Governing Vessel are important in Love-Shiatsu: GV 17, or Jade Pillow; GV 15; GV 14; GV 11, center of the fire of love; GV 4, the Door of Life; GV 3, a powerful arousal point; GV 2, the Valley of Delight; and GV 1, Lasting Strength.

GV 17, Jade Pillow, is where the impulse of passion flows into the brain, loving and rejuvenating and coursing through the cranial ocean to open the third eye (fig. 2.76).

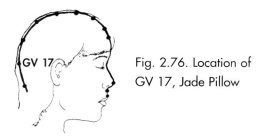

Fig. 2.76. Location of GV 17, Jade Pillow

GV 15 calms the mind, sending waves of relaxation through the nervous system, making it receptive to arousal (fig. 2.77).

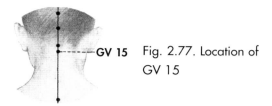

Fig. 2.77. Location of GV 15

Pressure applied to GV 14 sends a warm rush of spinal fluid up to the brain, generating excitement and warming the neck (fig. 2.78).

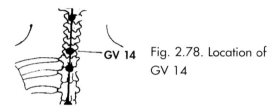

Fig. 2.78. Location of GV 14

GV 11, the center of the fire of love, is behind the heart, between the shoulder blades (fig. 2.79).

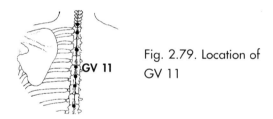

Fig. 2.79. Location of GV 11

GV 4, Ming Men or Door of Life, is the point where life enters at the moment of conception (fig. 2.80). It is a powerful arousal point, and aids male sexual stamina. It is also useful for relief of post-coital lower back pain.

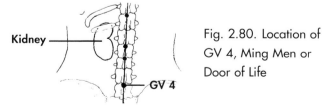

Fig. 2.80. Location of GV 4, Ming Men or Door of Life

GV 3, a powerful arousal point for both sexes, is just above the sacrum, at the back of the sexual center (fig. 2.81). Stimulation of this point helps in regulating menstruation in women and aids men in overcoming impotence and controlling wet dreams.

GV 2, Valley of Delight, is an arousal point (fig. 2.82).

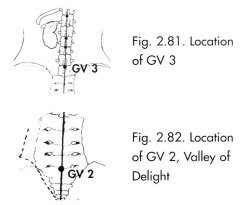

Fig. 2.81. Location of GV 3

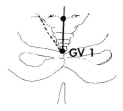

Fig. 2.82. Location of GV 2, Valley of Delight

Stimulation of GV 1, Lasting Strength, can send waves of electric pleasure coursing through the sacral bone, the sacred connection with the nerves of love (fig. 2.83).

Fig. 2.83. Location of GV 1, Lasting Strength

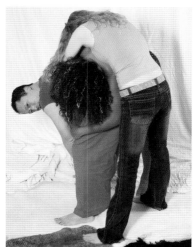

Fig. 2.84. Stretching the Governing Vessel is the same as stretching the spine. Just bend forward as far as you can and get a friend to help with his or her weight.

Conception Vessel: Yin Meridian

The Conception Vessel is the front channel of the Microcosmic Orbit (fig. 2.85). It begins at the very base of the being, the point called the Gate of Life and Death, from which energy pours at the moment of childbirth, also menstrual flow for women and ejaculation for men. This meridian connects the organs of conception (the Jade Stalk in men and the Yin Gate in women) with the Sperm Palace or Ovarian Palace, the navel center, solar plexus, heart center, and throat, thus combining the energies of love and sex, yang and yin, fire and water.

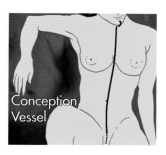

Fig. 2.85. Conception Vessel: yin meridian

The route of this channel tells its story: it runs from the Gate of Life and Death in the base chakra, up through the genitals, the belly, and the heart to the root of the tongue (fig. 2.86).

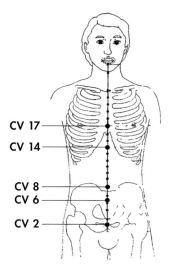

Fig. 2.86. Conception Vessel runs from the Gate of Life and Death in the base chakra, up through the genitals, the belly, and the heart to the root of the tongue.

CV 17
CV 14
CV 8
CV 6
CV 2

Two of the most powerful arousal points lie along the Conception Vessel. These energy vortexes should be approached with love, care, and respect. Prepare your lover with whole body Love-Shiatsu (see chapter 3), then—as you palm-step down the Nine Flowers—linger on CV 6 for a man and CV 2 for a woman.

CV 17, or Central Altar, also known as the Sea of Tranquillity, is the point for sharing true love (fig. 2.87). Connection here calms the mind, balances emotions, and calms the spirit of the heart.

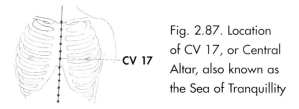

Fig. 2.87. Location of CV 17, or Central Altar, also known as the Sea of Tranquillity

CV 14, or Great Palace, is the gateway to the heart itself, which you can use to access the heart fire of your lover (fig. 2.88).

CV 8 is the Spirit's Palace Gate (fig. 2.89).

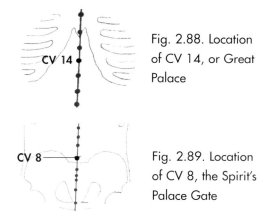

Fig. 2.88. Location of CV 14, or Great Palace

Fig. 2.89. Location of CV 8, the Spirit's Palace Gate

CV 6, the Sea of Chi, is the male sexual energy center (fig. 2.90). This most potent male arousal point also connects with the essence of the feminine, related to the feminine reproductive cycle. Clinical stimulation of this point helps with menstrual difficulties.

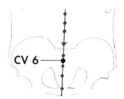

Fig. 2.90. Location of
CV 6, the Sea of Chi

CV 2 is the most potent feminine arousal point and also quite effective for men (fig. 2.91).

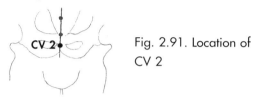

Fig. 2.91. Location of
CV 2

CV 1, the Gate of Life and Death, is so named because the retention of sexual energy is said to prolong life (fig. 2.92). Subtle use of CV 1 is arousing for both sexes, and is especially good for prolonging male orgasm. Clinical stimulation of this point helps with prevention and relief of prostate conditions.

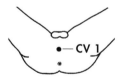

Fig. 2.92. Location of
CV 1, the Gate of Life
and Death

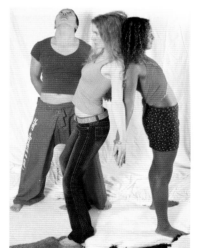

Fig. 2.93. Bend over
backward to stretch
Conception Vessel but
take care not to strain
your back. Get help!

Connection to Infinity

Connecting the Governing Vessel and the Conception Vessel in the act of love makes a channel of love energy flowing through the lovers, coursing up the back and down the front of both, fusing yin and yang, uniting their chakra energy centers in the flow of infinity (fig. 2.94).

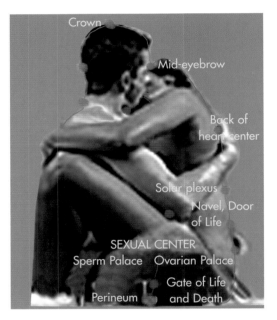

Fig. 2.94. Connecting the Governing Vessel and the Conception Vessel in the act of love makes a channel of love energy uniting the lovers' chakra energy centers in the flow of infinity.

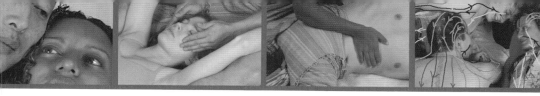

Whole Body Love-Shiatsu

Love-Shiatsu, over three thousand years old, is one of the most sexually exciting games in love-play. By following its teachings about the body's areas of arousal and using energy meridians as pathways for your hands, you can enhance your intimate connection with your lover and increase the chemistry of desire.

You can practice your Love-Shiatsu with a friend in order to get feedback about what feels really good, what maybe does not, how much pressure you should put here and there. Sensitivity comes easily: just notice how your partner responds to your touch. Anticipate arousal: agree how far you are both willing to go and decide on a stop signal if it gets too hot to handle.

PREPARATION FOR LOVE-SHIATSU

The person receiving the massage should lie on a floor mat, a narrow table, or a firm bed: flaccidity is no help inside or out. You can perform Love-Shiatsu without any lubricant, or you can use scented water or oil such as sesame oil. A good brisk hand-rub before you touch will energize your hands.

Atmospherics for Love

Make your bower beautiful, enticing, a place for pleasure. Feng shui your love life: make space around your love nest; have a picture of your beloved in the southwest corner, and a green plant in the east. Arrange things to please all the senses before starting your Love-Shiatsu:

- Candlelight and soft music, yes. Phones, no: off or silent, rings on mute.
- Fragrances of roses, musk, and ylang ylang.
- Aphrodisiac tidbits to tantalize taste buds: chocolate, strawberries, and bananas or cucumbers dipped in clove honey, mangos, peaches, plums, and cherries.
- If you like salads, try celery, mushrooms, red peppers, spinach, tomatoes, and watercress.
- Try using each other as a plate.
- And to drink? Try mead, a mildly alcoholic beverage made from honey. In Anglo-Saxon England newly-weds retired for a moon month to a flowery bower to live on nothing but love and mead: thus the word *honag monath* or "honeymoon."
- Dress in loose, light clothing, soft fabrics of red, pink, and purple. Sarongs don't get in the way; they let you reach all the love points and come off easily.

Prepare Your Lover

Lovers have always touched. It starts with a look, a gaze in each other's eyes. Then mind follows eye and hand follows mind (fig. 3.1).

Prepare your lover by first lightly tapping or patting and then stroking up and down the body. You don't have to follow the lines pictured exactly; they are just there to give you an idea of the flow of energy along the meridians (see fig. 3.2 on page 58).

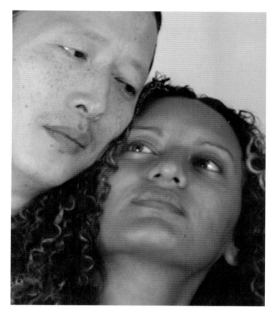

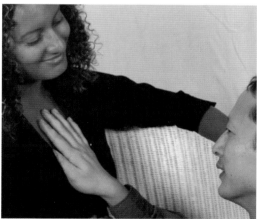

Fig. 3.1. A lover's touch begins with a look.

Tapping wakes up the nerves. How do you like to be woken up? Tap very gently on softer areas such as the belly and face, and not at all on breasts and genitals. Get feedback from your lover on how it feels: would they like a drum solo in some places, such as the sacrum and shoulder blades, or would they prefer tippy-toe tap?

Once the nerves are awake, they will be ready to be coaxed into action. Go from tapping to rubbing, not too hard, not too soft. Follow the meridian routes more or less, just to let them know you will be back. Continue to avoid the genitals, for now.

When you have tapped and rubbed, its time to tease: long languorous strokes along the channels, brushing close by your lover's genitals, using your hands to hint at what's ahead. Take your time with this stage, allowing your lover's arousal to build.

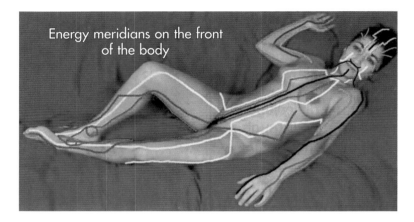

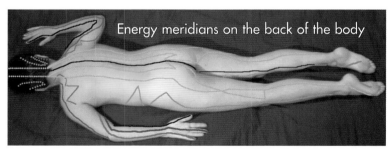

Fig. 3.2. Tap, rub, and stroke along the meridian pathways to prepare your lover for the full-body massage.

LOVE-SHIATSU NUMEROLOGY

Here are some numbers to guide you around the erotic landscape. The full-body shiatsu massage proceeds in five parts and stimulates thirty-three specific acupressure points to arouse the chemistry of desire in your lover. The parts of the massage are as follows:

Part One (steps 1–8): Ease your way down the back (fig. 3.3).

Part Two (steps 9–15): Make your way up the side (fig. 3.4).

Part Three (steps 16–23): Wander up and down the front (fig. 3.5).

Part Four (repeat steps 9–15): Turn your attention and loving caresses to the other side (fig. 3.6).

Part Five (steps 24–32): Then teasingly work your way down to heaven (fig. 3.7).

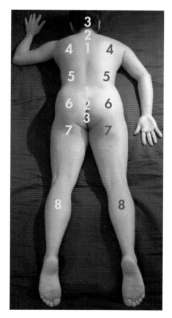

Fig. 3.3. Part One of the full-body massage moves down the back.

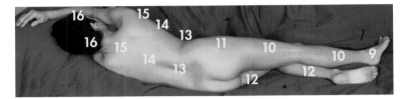

Fig. 3.4. Part Two of the full-body massage
moves up the right side.

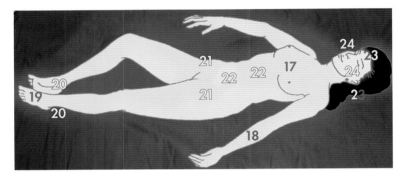

Fig. 3.5. Part Three of the full-body massage
wanders up and down the front.

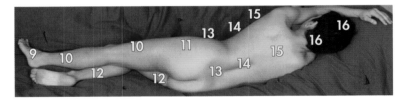

Fig. 3.6. Part Four of the full-body massage
moves up the left side.

The numbers superimposed over the photos on these pages show the step-by-step sequence of the massage. On the following pages you will see more specifically where you can place your hands, fingers, and thumbs to lay and light the fires. By following the simple hand-by-hand routine you will connect all the arousal points and give your partner a wonderful sensual experience.

The sequence and points of connection are shown to help you find your own way—no need to get too technical about it! If you are doing

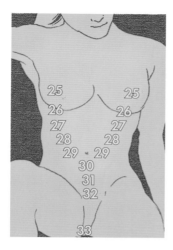

Fig. 3.7. Part Five of the full-body massage makes its way down to heaven.

it with sensitivity, care, and love, you are doing it right. Remember, it is a really good idea to ask your partner how it feels.

Be creative; enjoy your pleasures.

The Full-Body Shiatsu Love Massage

Part One: Moving Down the Back

The first three steps in Part One connect points on the Governing Vessel energy pathway running down the middle of the back (fig. 3.8).

Energize your hands by rubbing them together briskly before you begin.

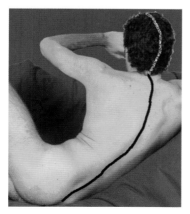

Fig. 3.8. The Governing Vessel energy pathway runs down the middle of the back.

Step 1

Connecting Fire and Water Using Points GV 11 and GV 3

Let your hands alight on points GV 11 behind the heart and GV 3 just above the sacrum, blending the heart love with sexual desire to harmonize fire and water, yin and yang (figs. 3.9 and 3.10).

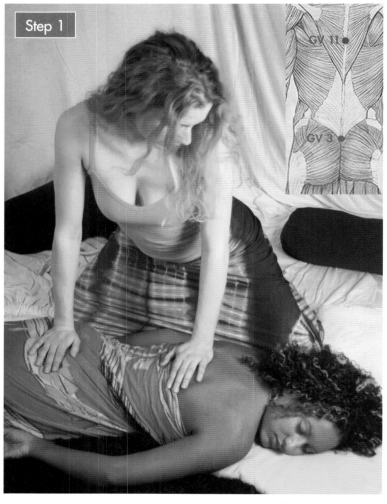

Fig. 3.9. Step 1 connects the fire energy of the heart center with the water energy of the kidney center.

Shiatsu Secret: Let your hands be still, resting on your lover. Feel the warmth. Close your eyes. Imagine both hands in a pool of warmth, surrounding and connecting them.

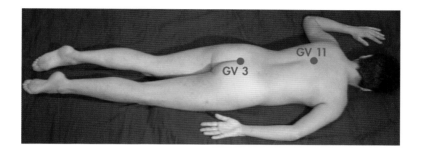

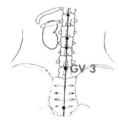

GV 3 is a powerful arousal point for both sexes, just above the sacrum, at the back of the sexual center.

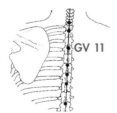

GV 11 is the center of the fire of love, behind the heart, between the shoulder blades.

Fig. 3.10. The location of points
GV 3 and GV 11 on the back

Step 2

Connecting the Valley of Delight and GV 14

Now let your hands rest on GV 14 at the base of the neck and GV 2 on the sacrum (figs. 3.11 and 3.12).

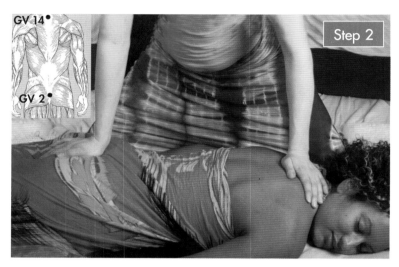

Fig. 3.11. In step 2 you begin to generate excitement and arousal by connecting GV 2 and GV 14.

Shiatsu Secret: Imagine the pool of warmth spreading out until it feels like you are touching your lover in only one place. When it feels like that to you, your lover too will feel as if you are touching in just one place, however far apart your hands may be.

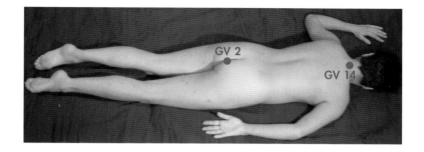

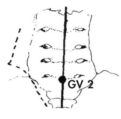

GV 2 Valley of Delight
arousal point

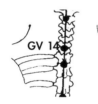

GV 14 sends a warm rush of
spinal fluid up to the brain,
generating excitement and
warming the neck.

Fig. 3.12. Location of points GV 2 and GV 14 on the back

Step 3

Connecting Heaven and Earth Using GV 17 and GV 1

Sliding along the river of love into realms above and below, connect the Gate of Heaven (GV 17) with the Door to Earth (GV 1) (figs. 3.13 and 3.14).

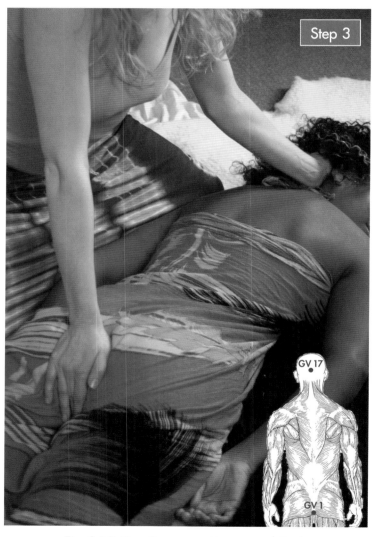

Fig. 3.13. Step 3 connects Heaven and Earth by connecting GV 17 and GV 1.

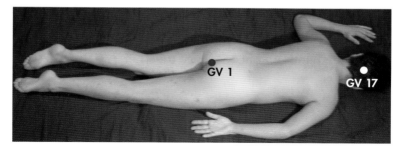

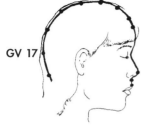

GV 17, Jade Pillow, where the impulse of passion flows into the brain, loving and rejuvenating and coursing through the cranial ocean to open the mid-eye.

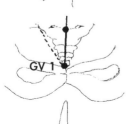

GV 1, Lasting Strength, where waves of electric pleasure course through the sacral bone, the sacred connection with the nerves of love.

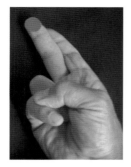

Put your index finger on top of your middle finger and use both to press these points.

Fig. 3.14. Location of points GV 1 and GV 17 on the back and instructions for how to press them

Step 4

Joining Two Fire Meridians—Heart Protector and Small Intestine

Place the middle of each palm (HP 8) on SI 11, found on each of your lover's shoulder blades (figs. 3.15 and 3.16). Listen carefully to the breath below and follow its rhythm; hands and heart dance together, courting lust.

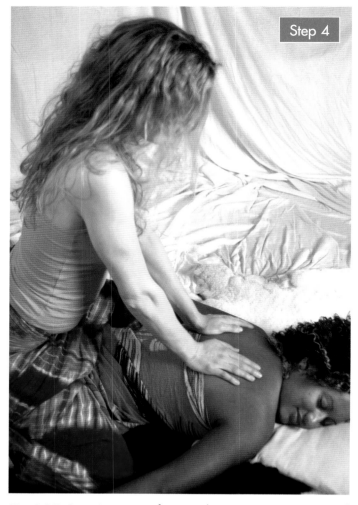

Fig. 3.15. Step 4 joins two fire meridians—Heart Protector and Small Intestine—to generate some heat.

Shiatsu Secret: Each time you move one hand, again imagine the pool of warmth connecting both your hands and the places you are touching on your lover's body.

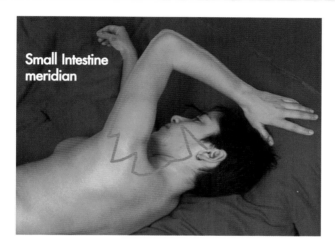

Small Intestine meridian

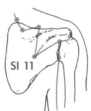

SI 11

SI 11 eases the shoulders with gentle palm or focused finger.

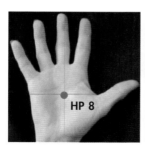

HP 8

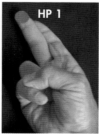

HP 1

Fig. 3.16. Massage the Small Intestine 11 point on the shoulder blade with Heart Protector 8 in the palm of the hand. You can also use HP 1 at the tip of the middle finger to put more focused pressure on SI 11.

Step 5

Connecting the Kidney Meridian to the Gate of Life and Death

Part your partner's legs with your knee, and place your thumbs on either side of the spine. Arousal energy starts to wake up and flow (figs. 3.17 and 3.18).

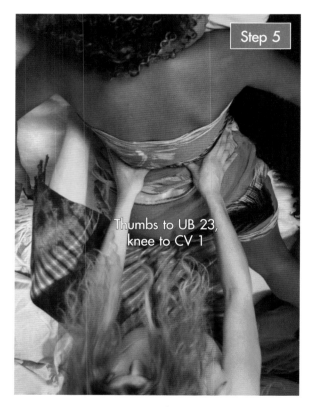

Fig. 3.17. Connecting UB 23, the Kidney connector point, and CV 1, the Gate of Life and Death, promotes arousal and sexual vitality.

Shiatsu Secret: Hold the vision of the pool of warmth each time you move your hands. Your lover will feel as if his or her whole body is being bathed in love and warmth. You are preparing for passion.

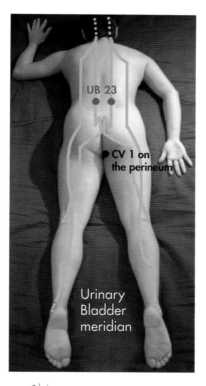

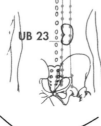

UB 23, the Kidney connector point, promotes sexual vitality for both sexes and enhances male stamina.

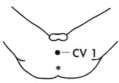

CV 1, the Gate of Life and Death

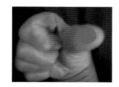

Use your thumb to press on UB 23.

Fig. 3.18. Location of points UB 23 and CV 1 and instructions for how to press them

Step 6

Spiral Massage of the Buttocks

Kneel between your partner's legs, move your hands to the buttocks, sending flashes of desire along the sides of the body. Starting at GB 30, spiral inward, rubbing the cheeks together to stimulate arousal (figs. 3.19 and 3.20).

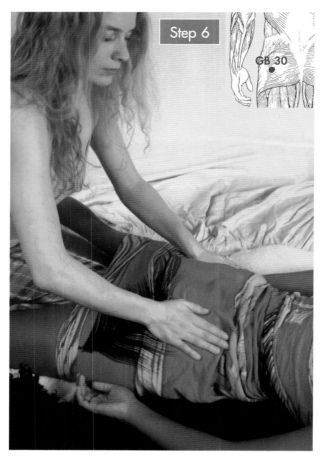

Fig. 3.19. Starting at GB 30, a spiral massage of the buttocks stimulates arousal.

More Secrets await discovery in the points of connection. Tune in to your partner's response to your every touch. Don't be afraid to ask: "How does this feel?" "Do you like it?" "Would you like more?"

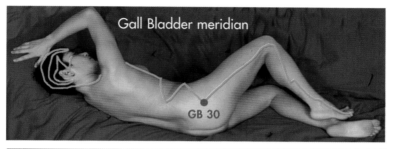

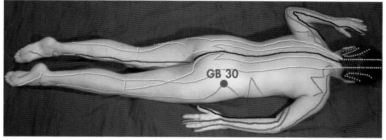

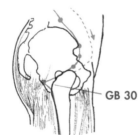

GB 30, Jumping Circle, starting point for a beautiful spiral massage around the buttocks

Fig. 3.20. Location of the Gall Bladder 30 point on the buttocks

Step 7

Joining HP 8 with UB 37 to Warm the Legs

Starting the tease, stay kneeling between the legs but move hands away from the erogenous zone. Stay on the Urinary Bladder meridian, though, pressing UB 37 on each leg with HP 8 in the palms of your hands (figs. 3.21 and 3.22). The Urinary Bladder meridian carries arousal messages through the whole energy body from head to toe.

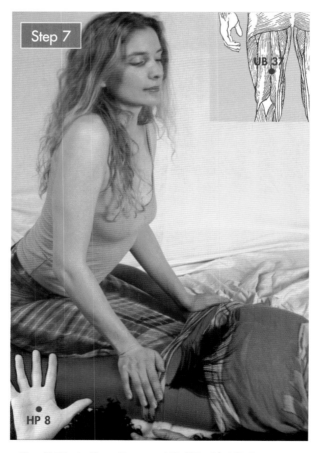

Fig. 3.21. In Step 7, press UB 37 with HP 8 to warm the legs and keep the arousal going.

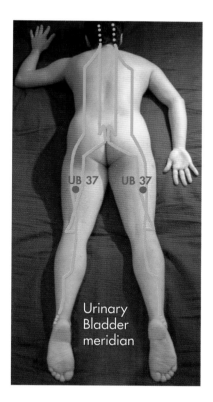

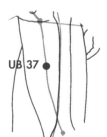

UB 37 warms the whole leg and sends the love signals both ways.

Fig. 3.22. Location of the UB 37 point on the back of the thigh

Steps 8 and 9

Connect to Your Lover's Sexual Essence at KD 1 and KD 3

A wealth of sexual connections are found on the feet. As you support your lover's foot on your pubic bone, site of CV 2, simultaneously press KD 1 on the ball of the foot, KD 3 on the inner ankle, and UB 60 on the outer ankle (figs. 3.23, 3.24, and 3.25). Feeling the strength of your partner's Achilles tendon can give an indication of sex drive.

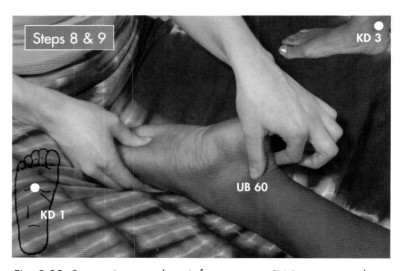

Fig. 3.23. Supporting your lover's foot on your CV 2, connect to his or her sexual essence at KD 1 and KD 3. Pinch the Achilles tendon at UB 60 to gauge your partner's libido.

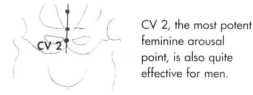

CV 2, the most potent feminine arousal point, is also quite effective for men.

Fig. 3.24. Location of Conception Vessel 2 at the pubic bone

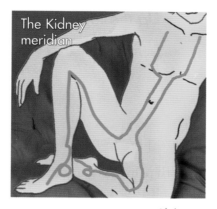

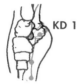

KD 1, Bubbling Spring, where you keep your feet on the ground

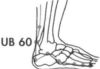

UB 60, Kunlun Mountain

KD 3, Great Stream, can be used to either stimulate or balance desire in both sexes.

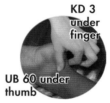

Pinching here gives a good idea of the strength of your partner's libido: the stiffer the stronger! This is also a useful point to press during labor.

Fig. 3.25. Location of KD 1 on the ball of the foot, KD 3 on the inner ankle, and UB 60 on the outer ankle

This completes Part One of the full-body massage. It's time to leave the back and move up your lover's right side.

☍ *Part Two: Moving Up the Right Side*

As you cruise with your palms, be aware of the slow soft bolts of desire.

Step 10

Generate Desire by Joining LV 9 and SP 6

> Using HP 8 on both palms, place your left hand on your partner's left leg at LV 9 on the inner thigh and your right hand on SP 6 (figs. 3.26 and 3.27).

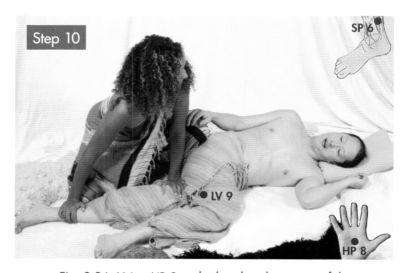

Fig. 3.26. Using HP 8 on both palms, be aware of the soft bolts of desire as you place your left hand on your partner's left leg at LV 9 on the inner thigh and your right hand on SP 6 above the ankle on the inside.

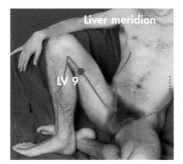

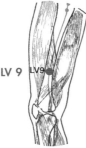

LV 9 is a subtle arousal point, situated on the pleasure muscles of the inner thigh approaching the sexual organs.

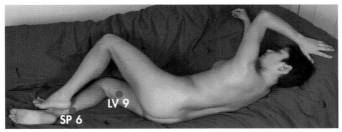

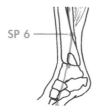

SP 6, Meeting of 3 Yin, is a versatile point, helpful for conditions of impotence, frigidity, and premature ejaculation.

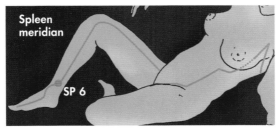

Fig. 3.27. Location of LV 9 and SP 6

Steps 11 and 12

Warming Your Lover's Urinary Bladder Meridian with Your Spleen Meridian

Move in for more close-contact work: straddle your CV 1 across your lover's Liver meridian and nestle his or her Urinary Bladder meridian with your Spleen meridian. Your thigh will be providing warmth to UB 36 in particular. Then use your elbow to apply pressure to the GB 30 point on his or her right buttock (figs. 3.28 and 3.29).

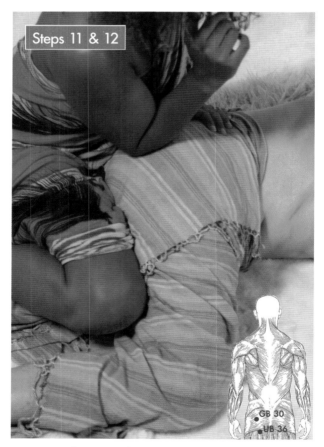

Fig. 3.28. Move in for more close-contact work and increasing warmth.

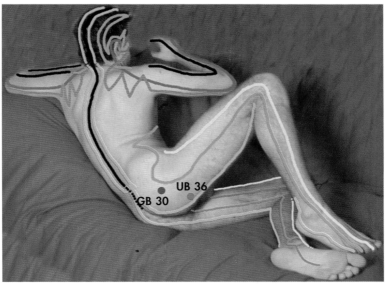

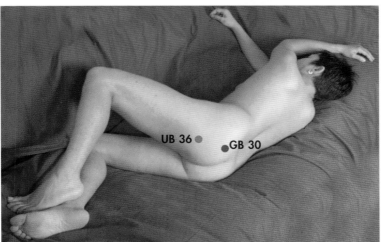

Fig. 3.29. Location of GB 30 and UB 36

Steps 13, 14, and 15

Connecting Your Lover's Door of Life and Spirit's Palace Gate

Press your leg against your lover's CV 1 and GV 2 while his or her buttock touches your CV 2. Connect your lover's GV 4, Door of Life, on the lower back and CV 8, the Spirit's Palace Gate, center front, by placing one hand on each (figs. 3.30 and 3.31). Stay in position long enough to feel total connection before continuing your seductive upward journey.

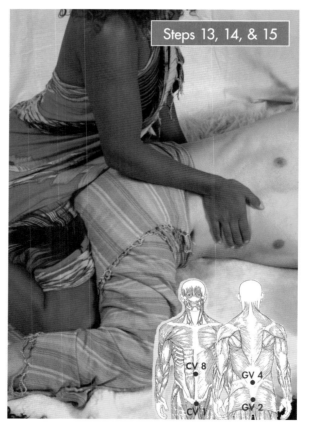

Fig. 3.30. Press your leg against your lover's CV 1 and GV 2 while his or her buttock touches your CV 2. Feel the electricity as you connect your lover's GV 4 on the lower back and CV 8, center front, by placing one hand on each.

Shiatsu Secret: The front-back connection between your hands reveals another secret—the pool of warmth becomes an electric charge.

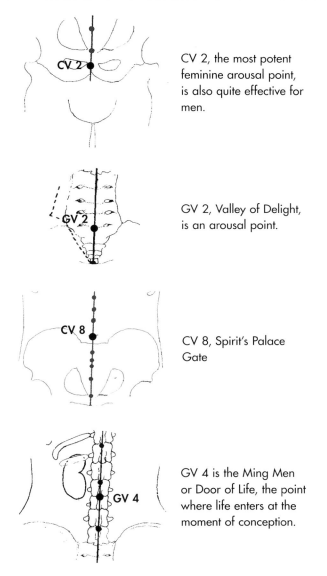

CV 2, the most potent feminine arousal point, is also quite effective for men.

GV 2, Valley of Delight, is an arousal point.

CV 8, Spirit's Palace Gate

GV 4 is the Ming Men or Door of Life, the point where life enters at the moment of conception.

Fig. 3.31. Location of CV 2, GV 2, CV 8, and GV 4

Step 16

Supporting GV 15 with HP 8 to Calm the Mind and Promote Relaxation

Gently support GV 15 at the base of your lover's skull with Heart Protector 8 in the palm of your hand to calm the mind and send waves of relaxation through the nervous system, making it receptive to arousal (figs. 3.32 and 3.33).

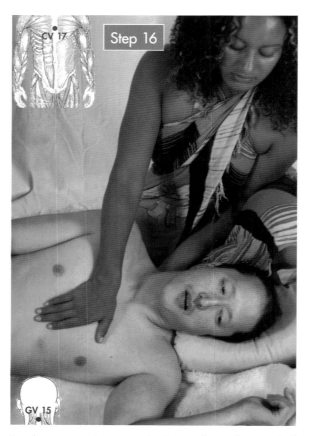

Fig. 3.32. Gently support GV 15 at the base of your lover's skull with HP 8 in the palm of your hand to send waves of relaxation through the nervous system to make it receptive. Then begin Part Three of the massage by placing your other palm on CV 17 in the center of the chest.

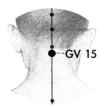

GV 15 calms the mind, sending waves of relaxation through the nervous system, making it receptive to arousal.

Fig. 3.33. Location of GV 15

This completes Part Two of the full-body Love-Shiatsu massage. However, you can smoothly continue with Part Three as you place your other palm on Conception Vessel 17 in the center of the chest while continuing to support Governing Vessel 15 at the base of the skull.

🌀 *Part Three: Wandering Up and Down the Front*

Step 17

Send Waves of Bliss through Your Lover
by Connecting GV 15 and CV 17

Use Heart Protector 8 in the palms of your hands to
connect Conception Vessel 17 in the center of the chest

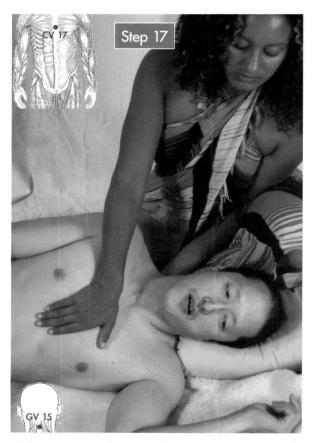

Fig. 3.34. While supporting GV 15 at the base of your lover's skull with HP 8
in the palm of your hand, begin Part Three of the massage by placing your
other palm on CV 17 in the center of the chest.

(figs. 3.34 and 3.35) and Governing Vessel 15 at the base of the skull; this will send waves of bliss throughout your lover's whole being, flooding both the physical and the energy bodies.

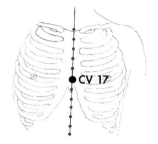

CV 17, Central Altar, is also known as the Sea of Tranquility and the point for sharing true love. Connection here calms the mind, balances emotions, and calms the spirit of the heart.

Fig. 3.35. Location of CV 17, Central Altar

Step 18

Stretch Your Lover to Release Sexual Tension

Stretches tend to disperse chi, so they are used infrequently in Love-Shiatsu. A stretch at this point, however, is well timed to ease the buildup of sexual tension likely to have arisen from the previous close connections. It is time for a breather. Even so, a nice straddle keeps up the interest, with your CV 1 sitting on your partner's LV 8 (figs. 3.36 and 3.37).

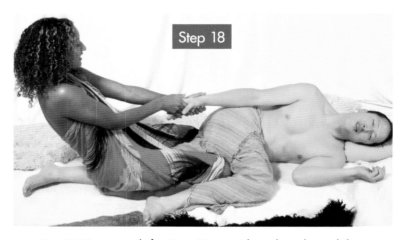

Fig. 3.36. A stretch for Step 18 provides a breather, while a nice straddle with your CV 1 on your partner's LV 8 keeps up the interest.

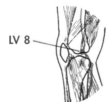

LV 8: regular massage of this point improves sexual function.

Fig. 3.37. Location of LV 8

Step 19

Connecting Your Lover's Bubbling Spring to Your Heart Fire

On reaching the feet, connect your lover's Bubbling Spring (KD 1) to your heart fire (CV 14). With one hand grasp LV 3 (on a woman) or LV 4 (on a man). With the other fondle UB 60 and KD 3. Meanwhile your partner's heel rests on your CV 2 (figs. 3.38, 3.39, and 3.40). Can this be the way to heaven? Yes, but it is just one of many. Hold for long enough to feel it, rhythmically rocking and rubbing.

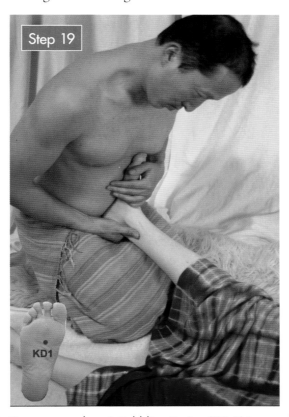

Fig. 3.38. Connect your lover's Bubbling Spring (KD 1) to your heart fire (CV 14). With one hand grasp LV 3 (on a woman) or LV 4 (on a man). With the other fondle UB 60 and KD 3. Meanwhile your partner's heel rests on your CV 2.

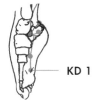

KD 1, Bubbling Spring, where you keep your feet on the ground, mostly

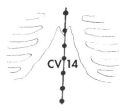

CV 14, Great Palace, is the gateway to the heart itself, the sovereign, which you can use to access the heart fire of your lover.

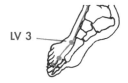

LV 3, Great Rushing, is particularly recommended for enhancing female sexual energy.

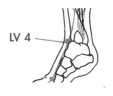

LV 4, Middle Barrier, is recommended for enhancing male sexual energy.

Fig. 3.39. Locations of KD 1, CV 14, LV 3, LV 4

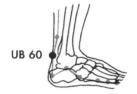

UB 60, Kunlun Mountain

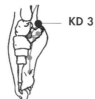

KD 3, Great Stream, can be used to either stimulate or balance desire in both sexes.

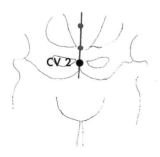

CV 2, the most potent feminine arousal point, is also quite effective for men.

Fig. 3.40. Locations of UB 60, KD 3, CV 2

Step 20

A Sensuous Foot-Belly Massage

Holding Bubbling Spring against your belly, rock in a circular rhythm so that you feel it where it matters and your lover feels it all over. Of course your lover thinks you are giving them the massage, but check out all your own sexy points covered by their feet: Stomach 21, Stomach 25, Liver 14, and Gall Bladder 24 (figs. 3.41 and 3.42). Meanwhile they feel the warmth of your belly, the movement of your muscles under their feet while your slow rocking rhythm vibrates up the legs to the hips.

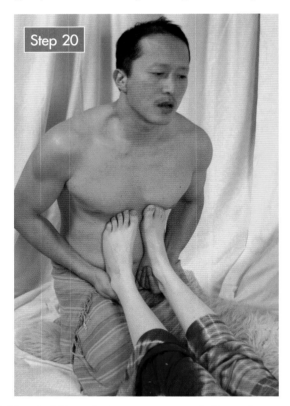

Fig. 3.41. Holding Bubbling Spring against your belly, rock in a circular rhythm so that you feel it where it matters and your lover feels it all over.

Shiatsu Secret: This foot-belly massage can be one of the most sensuous experiences you can share.

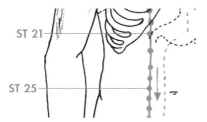

ST 21 is on the route of the Nine Flowers, the loving path down to heaven. It is very comforting and helps digest all the TLC.

ST 25, Heavenly Axis, awakens sensuality and opens the belly to pleasure.

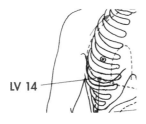

LV 14, Cyclic Gate, just below the underswell of the breast, is waiting to be rubbed.

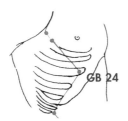

GB 24 warms the ribs and softens feelings of anxiety or indecision.

Fig. 3.42. Locations of Stomach 21, Stomach 25, Liver 14, and Gall Bladder 24

Step 21

Waking up SP 12, LV 12, and KD 11—A Trio of Loving Points in the Hips

As you hand-step up the body of your beloved, a trio of loving points lurk in both hips, waiting for you to find them and awaken them: SP 12, LV 12, and KD 11 (figs. 3.43 and 3.44).

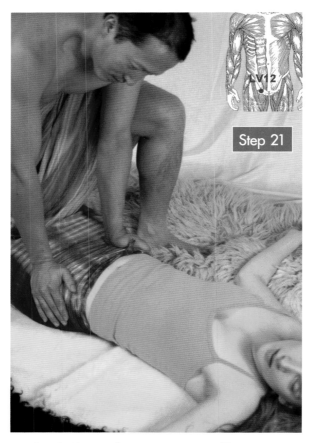

Fig. 3.43. Hand-step up to a trio of loving points in both hips waiting for you to find and awaken them.

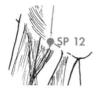

Gently stroking or simply holding
SP 12 with a still palm spreads
warmth and pleasure across the
genital area.

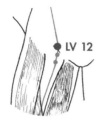

LV 12 increases energy circulation
and genital sensitivity.

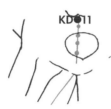

KD 11 helps with male arousal
difficulties.

Fig. 3.44. Locations of SP 12, LV 12, KD 11

Step 22

Connecting the Sea of Chi with the Sea of Tranquility

As well as offering a loving touch and lovely points of connection, placing your hands as shown (fig. 3.45) lets you move easily from one part of the body to another. Keep the connection with CV 6, the Sea of Chi, and CV 17, the Sea of Tranquility (or Central Altar) (fig. 3.46), while you think about where you want to go next, then move smoothly to the new position.

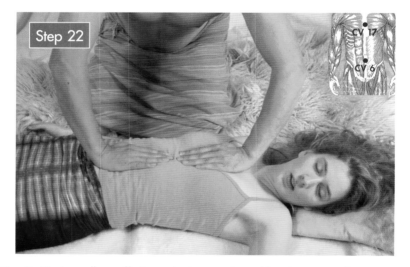

Fig. 3.45. As well as offering a loving touch and lovely points of connection, placing your hands as shown lets you move easily from one part of the body to another.

Shiatsu Secret: Remember to hold still until you feel the pool of warmth.

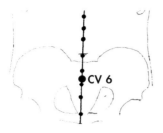

CV 6, the Sea of Chi, is the male sexual energy center. This most potent male arousal point also connects with the essence of the feminine.

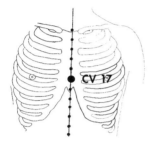

CV 17 or the Sea of Tranquility, also known as the Central Altar, is the point for sharing true love. Connection here calms the mind, balances emotions, and calms the spirit of the heart.

Fig. 3.46. Location of CV 6, Sea of Chi, and CV 17, Sea of Tranquility

Step 23

Connecting the Yin Tang and the Jade Pillow

Connecting the very special point, Yin Tang, with GV 17, Jade Pillow, creates a vortex of energy whirling through the brain. This is a magical connection: the point in the giver's palm, HP 8, is an extension of the heart chakra and can be used to convey the wave of love which then flows through the energy channels and floods the whole being (figs 3.47 and 3.48).

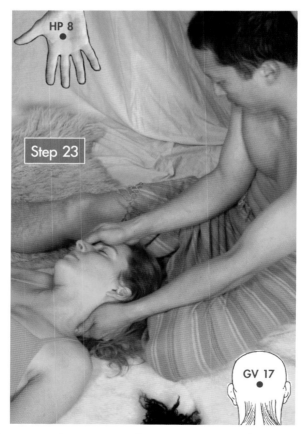

Fig. 3.47. Connecting the very special point, Yin Tang, with GV 17, Jade Pillow, creates a vortex of energy whirling through the brain. Then a wave of love flows through the energy channels and floods the whole being.

Shiatsu Secret: From the comfort of this position you can give the spiraling massage of Love-Shiatsu to many easily reachable parts.

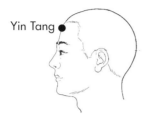

Yin Tang

The Yin Tang is a very special point that opens the third eye as a portal to the world of spirit. When lovers gaze into each other's eyes, each can see into the other's soul through this gateway.

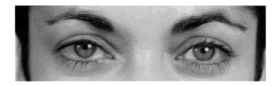

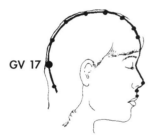

GV 17

GV 17, Jade Pillow, is where the impulse of passion flows into the brain, loving and rejuvenating and coursing through the cranial ocean to open the mid-eyebrow.

Fig. 3.48. Location of Yin Tang and GV 17, Jade Pillow

Step 24

Stroking the Flowers of the Elemental Organs in the Face

Time spent on the face is seldom wasted. Here bloom the flowers of the elemental organs: heart in the tongue, which you might leave for later, spleen in the lips, lung in the nose, kidney in the ears, and liver in the eyes. The meridians of Stomach, Gall Bladder, and Urinary Bladder begin on the face and Small Intestine, Large Intestine, and Triple Heater end here (figs. 3.49 and 3.50).

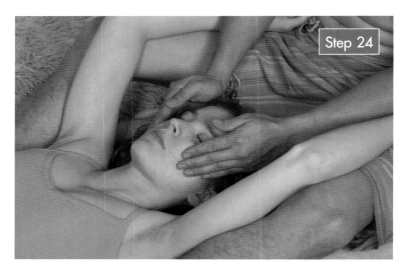

Fig. 3.49. Time spent on the face is seldom wasted. Here bloom the flowers of the elemental organs: heart in the tongue, spleen in the lips, lung in the nose, kidney in the ears, and liver in the eyes.

Shiatsu Secret: Don't be too surprised if by now you find your lover wanting to respond.

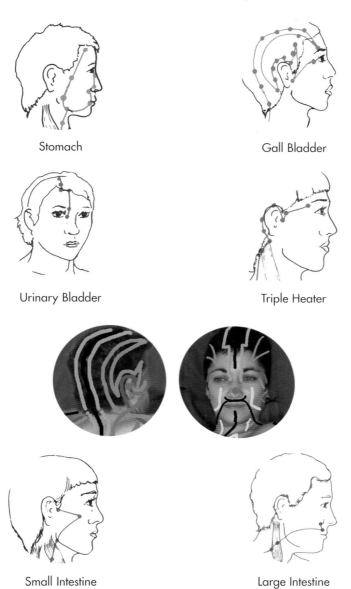

Fig. 3.50. Several meridians flow through the face:
Stomach, Gall Bladder, Urinary Bladder, Triple Heater,
Small Intestine, and Large Intestine.

🌀 Part Four: Moving Up the Left Side

You've done the back, one side, and the front of your lover. Now go back and do the other side, and make it a tease . . . returning, eventually, to . . . Stomach 17.

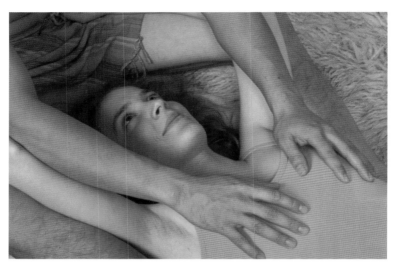

Fig. 3.51. Stomach 17, Breast Palace, is the starting point
for the beautiful and sensual Nine Flowers Massage—part 5 of the
Full-Body Shiatsu Love Massage that follows.

❂ Part Five: Moving Down to Heaven

The nine steps of Part Five comprise the Nine Flowers Massage (fig. 3.52).

NOW SLOW DOWN
DOWN
DOWN
Down

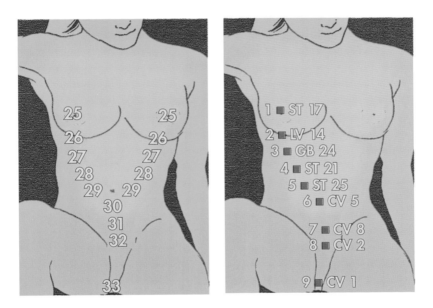

Fig. 3.52. The Nine Flowers are the focus of Steps 25–33.

Step 25

The First Flower, Breast Palace, Harmonizes Heart and Mind

The First Flower is ST 17, Breast Palace, a strong feminine arousal point that nurtures, soothes, and harmonizes heart and mind in both sexes (figs. 3.53 and 3.54).

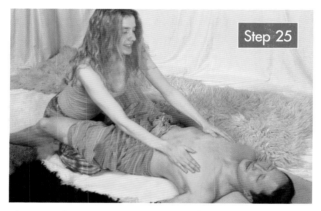

Fig. 3.53. The First Flower is ST 17, Breast Palace, a strong feminine arousal point that nurtures, soothes, and harmonizes heart and mind in both sexes.

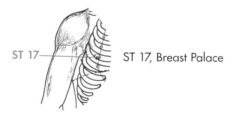

ST 17, Breast Palace

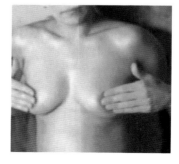

Fig. 3.54. Location of ST 17, Breast Palace

Step 26

The Second Flower, Cyclic Gate, Welcomes Your Caress

The Second Flower is LV 14, Cyclic Gate, just below the underswell of the breast. It is just waiting to be rubbed (figs. 3.55 and 3.56).

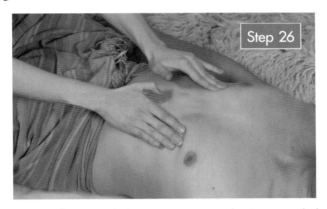

Fig. 3.55. The Second Flower is LV 14, Cyclic Gate, just below the underswell of the breast, and it is waiting to be rubbed.

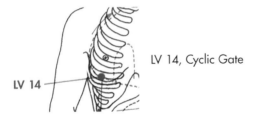

LV 14, Cyclic Gate

LV 14

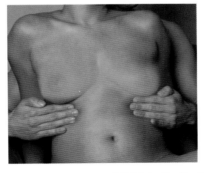

Fig. 3.56. Location of LV 14, Cyclic Gate

Step 27

The Third Flower, GB 24, Calms Anxiety

The Third Flower, GB 24, warms the ribs and softens feelings of anxiety or indecision (figs. 3.57 and 3.58).

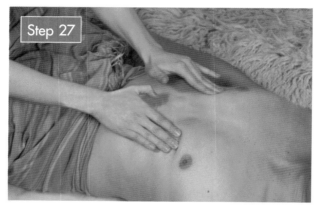

Fig. 3.57. The Third Flower, GB 24, warms the ribs and softens feelings of anxiety or indecision.

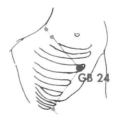

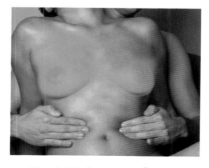

Fig. 3.58. Location of GB 24

Step 28

The Fourth Flower, ST 21, Digests All the Love

The Fourth Flower is ST 21: wandering down toward heaven, digesting all the love (figs. 3.59 and 3.60).

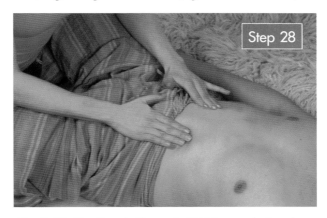

Fig. 3.59. The Fourth Flower is ST 21: wandering down to heaven, digesting all the love.

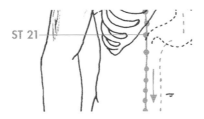

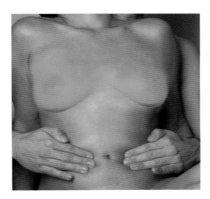

Fig. 3.60. Location of ST 21

Step 29

The Fifth Flower, Heavenly Axis, Awakens Sensuality

The Fifth Flower is ST 25, Heavenly Axis, which awakens sensuality and opens the belly to pleasure (figs. 3.61 and 3.62).

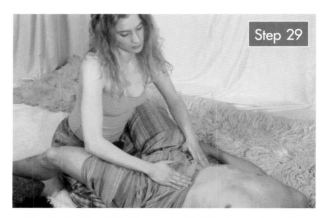

Fig. 3.61. The Fifth Flower is ST 25, Heavenly Axis, which awakens sensuality and opens the belly to pleasure.

ST 25

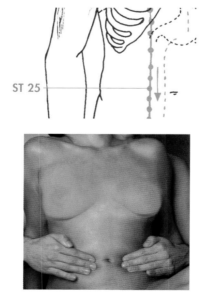

Fig. 3.62. Location of ST 25, Heavenly Axis

Step 30

The Sixth Flower, CV 6, Connects Male Arousal and Feminine Essence

The Sixth Flower is CV 6, the Sea of Chi, the male sexual energy center (figs. 3.63 and 3.64). This most potent male arousal point also connects with the essence of the feminine, related to the feminine reproductive cycle. Clinical stimulation of this point helps with menstrual difficulties.

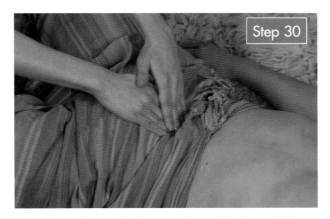

Fig. 3.63. The Sixth Flower is CV 6, the Sea of Chi, the male sexual energy center, which also connects with the essence of the feminine.

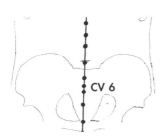

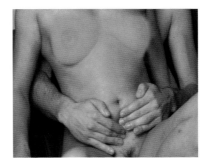

Fig. 3.64. Location of CV 6, the Sea of Chi

Step 31

The Seventh Flower, CV 3, Approaches Heaven (figs. 3.65 and 3.66).

The Seventh Flower is CV 3.

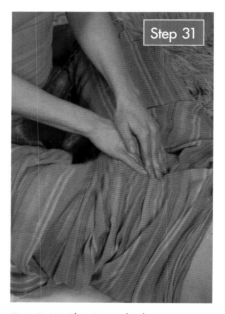

Fig. 3.65. The Seventh Flower, CV 3, moves closer to heaven.

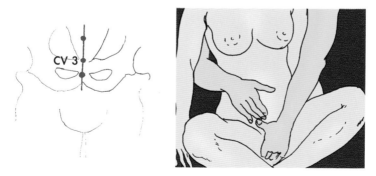

Fig. 3.66. Location of CV 3

Steps 32 and 33

The Eighth and Ninth Flowers, CV 2 and CV 1, Take You into Heaven

The Eighth Flower is CV 2, the most potent feminine arousal point, which is also quite effective for men. And the Ninth Flower is CV 1, the Gate of Life and Death, so named because the retention of sexual energy is said to prolong life (figs. 3.67 and 3.68). Subtle use of CV 1 is arousing for both sexes, and is especially good for prolonging male orgasm.

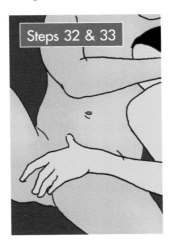

Fig. 3.67. Connect CV 2 and CV 1 to arrive in heaven.

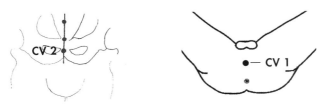

Fig. 3.68. Location of CV 2 and CV 1

After exchanging Love-Shiatsu, open to your creativity. Try tongue instead of hand, for instance . . .

Let the power of points, meridians, and elements inspire you!

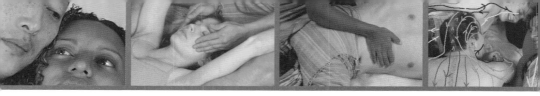

Self-Shiatsu:
Care and Maintenance

Self-Shiatsu that is directed to the specific pleasure points and love meridians of the body helps to keep your sexual energy alive, even when you are not having sex (figs. 4.1 and 4.2).

These massage techniques help both men and women to clear blockages in the chi flow while directing energy and blood into the sexual center. They will aid your awareness and care of the muscles that contribute to your strength and juice. To avoid confusion, the exercises for women and men are given in separate sections, followed by some for both.

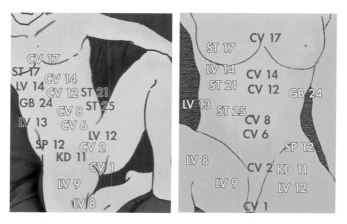

Fig. 4.1. Pressure points on the front of the body

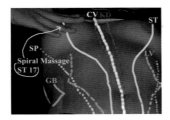

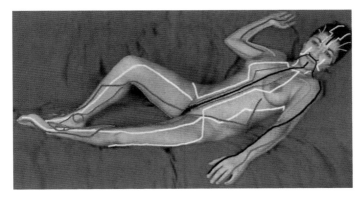

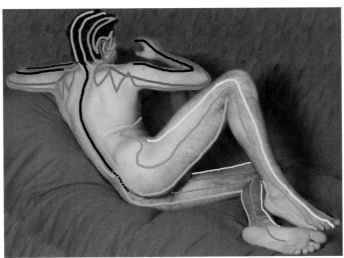

Fig. 4.2. Self-Shiatsu that is directed to the specific pleasure points and love meridians of the body helps to keep your sexual energy alive, even when you are not having sex.

EXERCISES FOR WOMEN

 ## Breast Massage

Massaging the breasts will enhance your arousal and enjoyment, help to keep your breasts healthy, and ease menstrual difficulties (the same meridian runs through nipples and ovarian tubes). As you do this exercise, combine the chi stimulated in the breasts with the additional energy of each successive gland, drawing it back to the breasts as the energy of each is activated. Think of the breasts as melting pots for the combined ingredients of chi from all of your glands.

1. Begin in a seated position, either naked or with a shawl or towel over your shoulders. You should feel a firm pressure against the vagina. To achieve this, place a rolled up towel between your legs.
2. Warm the hands by rubbing them together as you inhale, and press the tongue against the roof of the mouth.
3. Use the three middle fingers on each breast to circle outward from the nipples, and then inward again. Move your right hand clockwise, and your left hand counterclockwise, then reverse (36 times in each direction). Direct the chi accumulated in the breasts to the glands—from the pituitary down to the ovaries—and then bring it back to the breasts (fig. 4.3).

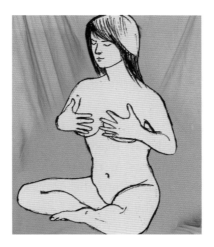

Activate the endocrine glands by massaging the area one and a half inches around the nipples.

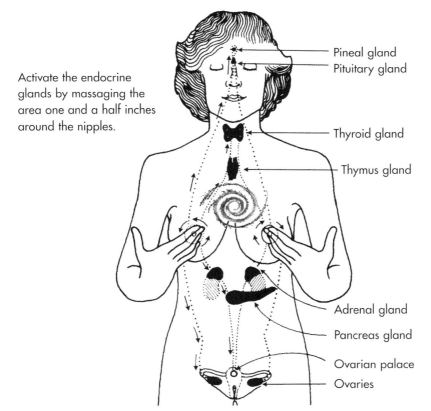

Pineal gland
Pituitary gland

Thyroid gland

Thymus gland

Adrenal gland

Pancreas gland

Ovarian palace
Ovaries

Fig. 4.3. Circulating the activated chi

Massage of the Ovaries and Uterus

This massage will increase your arousal and enjoyment, help to keep your reproductive organs healthy and free of stagnation, and ease menstrual difficulties.

1. After completing the breast massage, wait a few moments as the breast energy accumulates in the nipples, and then direct the energy flow directly down into the ovaries. Pause, and feel the accumulated energy in the ovaries.
2. Place each hand over its respective ovary at a hand's breadth below the navel on each side of the abdomen, and massage the ovaries 36 times in both directions as you did with the breasts (fig. 4.4).

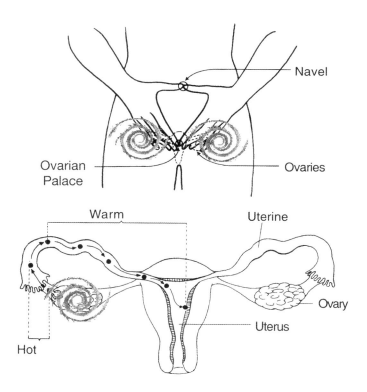

Fig. 4.4. Massage the ovaries, circling 36 times in both directions.

Internal Egg Exercise for Women

Jade eggs were used in the Imperial Court of ancient China for pleasure and health. Taoist women used them to strengthen the sexual region, thereby increasing both the sexual energy and life-force energy that was available to them. The Internal Egg exercise enables the practitioner to experience intensified pleasure and a strengthened grip. Regular practice of this exercise also enhances internal health by restoring and revitalizing the reproductive organs, harmonizing menstruation, and relieving symptoms of imbalance such as endometriosis (fig. 4.5).

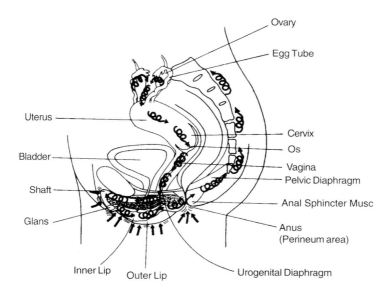

Fig. 4.5. Energy circulation in the female reproductive system

A stone egg is inserted into the vagina and then moved up and down the vaginal canal. This internal workout increases the strength of the lower abdomen and aids in gaining control over many of the involuntary muscles in the same area.

Eggs made of jade or obsidian are recommended because they

are sturdy, smooth, and non-porous. Wooden eggs, or any eggs with painted or chemical finishes, should be avoided. The egg should be drilled to accommodate a string passed through its center; the string makes it easy to remove the egg and also to apply internal pressure. These eggs are available through the Universal Tao.

The Internal Egg Exercise has five parts.

❷ Part One: Prepare Your Egg and Yourself

Before first use, boil your egg for about 20 minutes to dissolve the wax coating that protected it during shipping, and in case of possible handling by others.

1. Wash your egg in warm water before and after each practice. Soaking it in a solution of tea tree or grapefruit seed oil in water is also an option for afterward.
2. Insert the string into the hole in the egg and pull it through (fig. 4.6). Tie a knot in the string to prevent slipping.

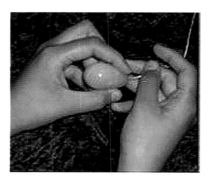

Fig. 4.6. Insert the string into the hole in the egg and pull it through.

3. Rub your hands vigorously to warm them and then massage your breasts, then your belly, mound of Venus, perineum, and genitals (fig. 4.7). Also give loving attention to your groin and inner thighs. Feel the warm loving energy open and melt away any tension, pain, or blockages, and start internal lubrication.

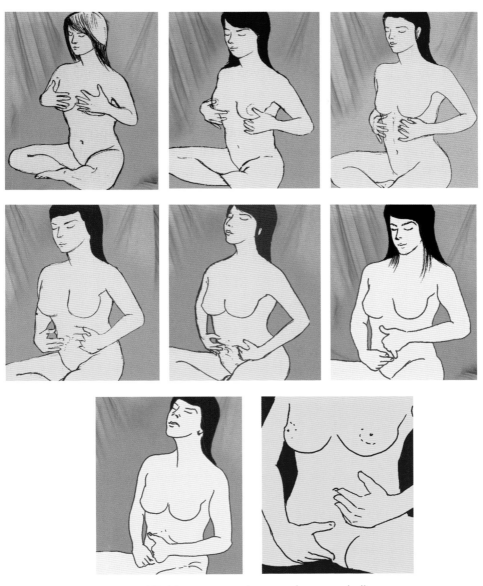

Fig. 4.7. Massage your breasts, then your belly,
mound of Venus, perineum, and genitals.

⟳ *Part Two: Insert the Egg*

Once you have sufficiently stimulated the breasts and the clitoris, warm, moist vaginal secretions will indicate that the body is ready for the egg to be inserted. If you like, use a non-toxic gel before insertion.

1. Gently place the egg, thicker end first, inside the inner labia and move it in slow circles until you feel it rest in a comfortable angle (fig. 4.8). Remember to take slow, deep breaths. Apply gentle pressure on the egg with your hand to encourage it to move into the vagina.

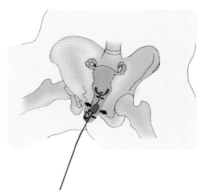

Fig. 4.8. Insert the egg into the vagina.

2. Gently feel the inner labia "sip" or "suck" the egg as you inhale, and feel the vagina "yawn" or open as you exhale. (This takes time to feel, so begin with simply smiling and imagining this.)
3. Continue the sipping exercise and add a gentle pelvic rock: rock your tailbone toward the ceiling as you inhale and press it into the floor as you exhale.
4. Tightly squeeze the egg as you inhale and push down/out as you exhale. The egg will move "in and out." Do this with or without the pelvic rock.

Value your own inner knowing and wisdom. If a practice doesn't feel right, experiment to create a special version for yourself.

☯ *Part Three: Basic Practice*

As you become more familiar with inserting the egg, you can increase the suction used to get it in. This practice can be done lying down (no gravity), seated, or standing.

1. Imagine breathing in to the ovaries. Focus your mind on your sexual energy. Visualize bringing the energy down through the uterus to the clitoris and holding it there.
2. Gently and slowly pull on the string and contract your vaginal muscles to keep the egg inside. With practice you can apply stronger pulls. Vary the angle of pull and observe the different sensations as the egg presses on different internal parts (fig. 4.9).

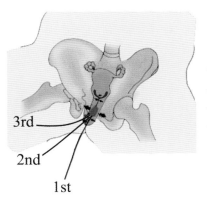

3rd

2nd

1st

Fig. 4.9. Three sections of the vaginal canal. Vary the angle of pull and observe the different sensations as the egg presses on different internal parts.

3. Isolate and slowly contract the muscle groups that close the vagina (as if stopping urination). Squeeze and release several times and feel the buildup of internal sensation.
4. Experiment with squeezes and angles of pull until satisfied.

🜨 *Part Four: Advanced Practices*

Once you are comfortable with the basic practice, you may want to try the following advanced practices. Between each exercise rub your hands warm, massage your belly/ovaries, and bring your hands up to your heart center and massage around the breasts in both directions.

1. For strengthening: while lying on your back, inhale and squeeze the genitals/egg and press your pelvis as high off the floor as possible, then exhale and relax/melt vertebrae back down to the floor.
2. Try the "Windshield Wiper": open your legs a little as you flex both feet simultaneously and keep them flexed the whole time. Rotate the legs away from each other and squeeze the buttocks, then rotate inward until your big toes touch. Feel the front and back of the genitals work.
3. Seated Practice: grab the egg with the genitals as you inhale and then relax as you exhale. Grip the egg with the genitals and move it up and down (fig. 4.10). Keep breathing slowly and smiling. Pull up and squeeze as you inhale, push down as you exhale. The egg will move up and down, but do not let it go out completely.

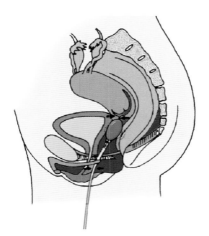

Fig. 4.10. The egg at the upper end of the vaginal canal

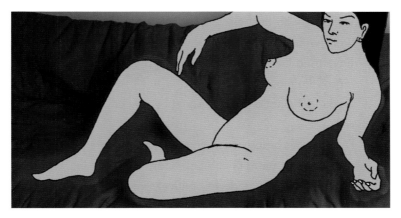

Fig. 4.11. Lie down and relax before gently withdrawing the egg.

Part Five: Removing the Egg

Lie down and relax for ten or fifteen minutes before gently withdrawing the egg (fig. 4.11).

1. Remove the egg by contracting the vaginal muscles to expel it. At first, it may help to squat or lift one leg on a short chair.

Important Hints for Practicing the Internal Egg Exercise

- Important: Rest after each exercise. If you feel any discomfort, massage the area with loving hands.
- Keep Smiling! Smiling helps keep the sexual energy in the body, allowing you to cultivate more and more energy without losing it.
- If you do not have a lot of time to do the practice, just keep the egg inserted as you move around the house, or out if you feel comfortable.
- If you are not lubricated enough, massage your nipples and/or use a lubricant of your choice with the egg.
- If you have difficulty holding the egg in at first, try

sleeping with it inserted. The genitals will continue to work with the egg as you sleep. Many women who have tried this have reported vivid dreams and a firming of the muscles.

- If you feel emotional or experience any pain, stop and rest.
- Five minutes a day of practice will create more positive results than one hour a week. Consistency is the key. Think of it as a wonderful, rejuvenating program.
- It is recommended that you rest from your practice while menstruating. Use your own discretion.
- Do not use an egg if you have an I.U.D.

EXERCISES FOR MEN

Generally men tend to touch their genital area on two occasions: to urinate or have sex, either alone or with someone else. Genital self-shiatsu is healthy as well as fun: it can increase blood flow to the penis, prevent stagnation in the testes and seminal ducts, and prevent deposit of the calcified salts that can lead to prostate conditions in later life.

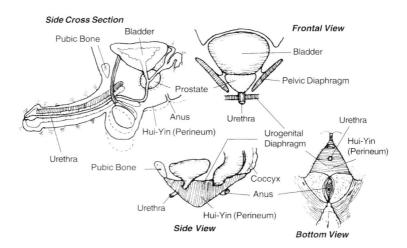

Fig. 4.12. The male genital area

Warming Up the Jade Stalk

Warming up the Jade Stalk by rolling it between your palms stimulates blood flow. Roll stalk between palms, gently at first then faster and more vigorously as if rubbing wood to make fire (fig. 4.13).

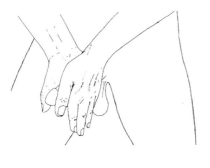

Fig. 4.13. Warming up the Jade Stalk

 ## Massage of the Dragon Pearls

Massage of the Dragon Pearls stretches the seminal ducts and prevents stagnation.

1. Rub your hands to warm them, then use them to warm the Dragon Pearls.
2. Gently pinch the scrotum above the right testicle with the right hand and above the left testicle with the left hand as shown (see fig. 4.14 on page 126). Pull outward and stretch.
3. Gripping the Dragon Pearls with your thumbs above and other fingers below, manipulate them between palms and fingers.
4. Place your left thumb on the top of your left testicle and the pinkie, fourth, third, and second fingertips of your left hand on the bottom. Hold the right testicle with the right hand in the same manner. Use your thumbs to gently press on each testicle. Then use your thumbs to massage around the testicles 36 times clockwise, and 36 times counterclockwise.

5. Continue to hold your left testicle in the same manner. At the same time, grasp the Jade Stalk firmly with your right hand. Pull the testicle to the left and the Jade Stalk to the right to give a good stretch (fig. 4.14 right).

6. Repeat, while holding the right testicle with the right hand pulling the Jade Stalk to the left.

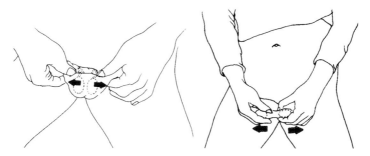

Fig. 4.14. Massage of the Dragon Pearls

 Stretching the Stalk

These exercises charge the sex organs with chi for increased strength and length, stimulate the meridians to prevent energy stagnation, and aid in detoxification. Before beginning, warm both hands by rubbing them together.

1. Encircle the base of the penis with the thumb and forefinger, as all of the fingers encircle the scrotum and surround the testicles.

2. Pull downward in a circular motion 9 to 36 times clockwise and then counterclockwise (fig. 4.15, upper).

3. Use the thumbs and index fingers of both hands to hold the base of the penis from the sides. Massage the penis along three lines as shown (fig. 4.15, lower left). Begin with the left line, using the left thumb and index finger to massage from the base of the penis to the tip and back. Then use the right thumb and index finger to massage the right line in the same manner.

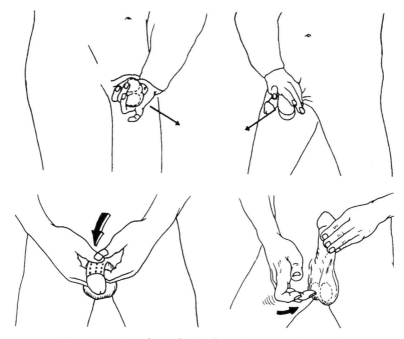

Fig. 4.15. Stretching the Stalk and tapping the Pearls

4. Next place both thumbs and index fingers on the middle line at the base, and massage down to the glans and back. Massage all three lines, counting up and down as one time, up to 36 times.

Tapping the Pearls

1. While holding the Jade Stalk up with the left hand, use the finger-tips of the right hand to lightly tap the right testicle. Tap in sets of 6, 7, or 9. Exhale, rest, and draw the energy up the spine (fig. 4.15 lower right).
2. Change hands and repeat with the left testicle.

EXERCISES FOR BOTH MEN AND WOMEN

Solo Exercises

 ### Bum Squeezing

The simple exercise of squeezing your buttocks together works to tone muscles and increase thrust (fig. 4.16).

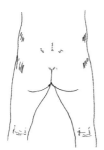 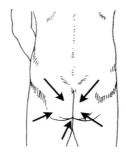 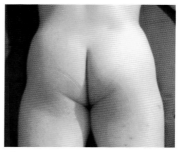

Fig. 4.16. Bum squeezing

 ### Focused Abdominal Breathing Exercise

Air = Energy: the more you can take in with least effort, the more you can put out.

1. Begin by breathing in, drawing the air into the abdomen. Make your chest hollow and drop the diaphragm down. You will feel pressure inside your abdomen, which will begin to protrude on all sides in a rounded shape (fig. 4.17).
2. As you exhale, draw your diaphragm up and squeeze in the abdomen to force the breath out of your nose.

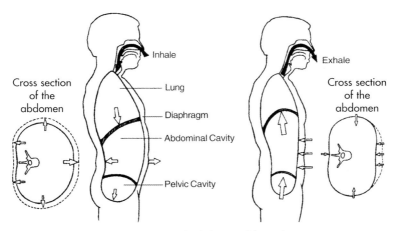

Fig. 4.17. Focused abdominal breathing

Mutual Exercises

 ### Massaging the Perineum

For men, massaging the perineum, particularly after ejaculation, keeps the prostate flexible and toned by preventing the deposit of calcified salts which can lead to unhealthy prostate conditions in later life (fig. 4.18). It's good to do it yourself and even more fun to have it done.

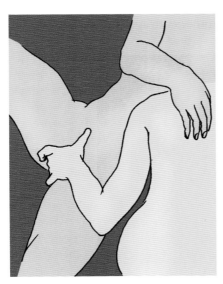

Fig. 4.18. For men, massaging the perineum, particularly after ejaculation, keeps the prostate flexible and toned.

For women, massaging ovaries, uterus, and perineum keeps strong, healthy energy flowing through the organs and meridians (fig. 4.19). Both do-it-yourself and sharing are effective and enjoyable.

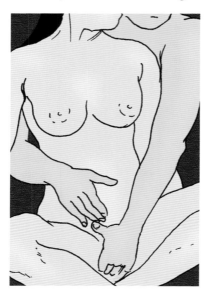

Fig. 4.19. For women, massaging ovaries, uterus, and perineum keeps strong, healthy energy flowing through the organs and meridians.

Breast Massage from a Friend

Breast massage from a friend gets right to the point (fig. 4.20). It's very important to give guidance and encourage sensitivity.

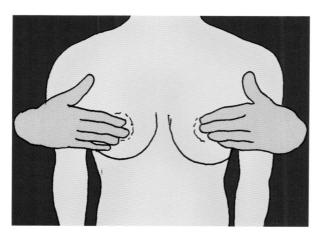

Fig. 4.20. Breast massage

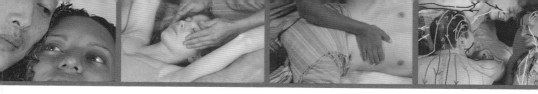

Compatibility: Marriages Made in Heaven

How do you and your lover suit each other? Do you get along well? Are you stormy or affectionate? Play buddies or committed partners?

Your compatibility is influenced by the following:

- When you were born and your resulting place in the Taoist zodiac
- Your nature, which is affected by how you live your life
- Your sexual interaction

You were each born as one of the twelve animals in the Taoist zodiac. Some of these animals are friends, others rivals, and some just get along without being especially friendly or competitive. By becoming aware of which animals play in your garden and how they interact, you will learn how to harmonize astrological imbalances.

Each of us is composed of all five elements but in the course of life, one will have become more predominant, determining how we respond to situations in the moment. Some elements support each other, while others control or regulate. A closer look at the relationships among the elements within you can help you harmonize imbalances in your relationships with other human beings.

One of you might have a stronger sexual appetite. It is likely that one of you becomes aroused more quickly. You may even prefer to play at different times of the day or night. You will see how you can smooth out the differences to make your loving more pleasurable and intense.

BIRTH YEARS

Our birth year tells us our animal in the Taoist medicine wheel. In the Chinese calendar the year starts in February, so if you are a January child put yourself in the previous year. (Chinese New Year is based on the lunar calendar so does vary from year to year, but February 4 is a good median guide.)

In the table below, the years are color-coded in pairs according to their element: red is fire; yellow is earth; black (for white) is metal; blue is water; and green is wood. Yang and yin exist within each element: the first of each color pair is the yang year, the second the yin year.

BIRTH YEARS

Rat	1936	1948	1960	1972	1984	1996	2008
Ox	1937	1949	1961	1973	1985	1997	2009
Tiger	1938	1950	1962	1974	1986	1998	2010
Rabbit	1939	1951	1963	1975	1987	1999	2011

Dragon	1940	1952	1964	1976	1988	2000	2012
Snake	1941	1953	1965	1977	1989	2001	2013
Horse	1942	1954	1966	1978	1990	2002	2014
Sheep	1943	1955	1967	1979	1991	2003	2015
Monkey	1944	1956	1968	1980	1992	2004	2016
Rooster	1945	1957	1969	1981	1993	2005	2017
Dog	1946	1958	1970	1982	1994	2006	2018
Pig	1947	1959	1971	1983	1995	2007	2019

FRIENDS AND RIVALS

Some animals get along with each other and others compete. The Triangles of Friends (fig. 5.1) show who your two best friends are, the Circle of Rivals (fig. 5.2) identifies your opponent.

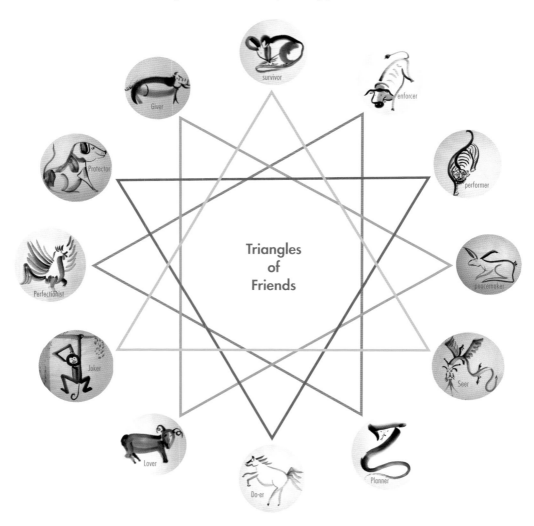

Fig. 5.1. Find your two best friends.

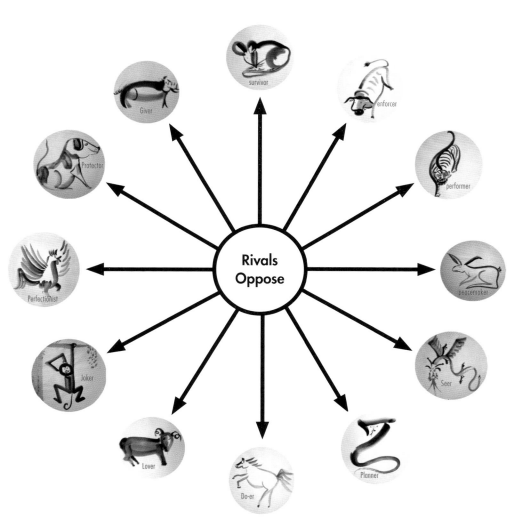

Fig. 5.2. Who has opposing energy?

BIRTH TIME AND THE ELEMENTS

In determining rivalry, the time of your birth also matters. For example, if you were born in the Year of the Tiger, your rival would be the Monkey. But if either of you were born in the other's month or hour, this would soften the rivalry, due to favorable elemental combinations. In the tables below showing the months and hours and their corresponding elements, red is fire, yellow is earth, black (for white) is metal, blue is water, and green is wood.

ANIMALS, BIRTH MONTHS, AND ELEMENTS

Rat	mid November to mid December
Ox	mid December to mid January
Tiger	mid January to mid February
Rabbit	mid February to mid March
Dragon	mid March to mid April
Snake	mid April to mid May
Horse	mid May to mid June
Sheep	mid June to mid July
Monkey	mid July to mid August
Rooster	mid August to mid September
Dog	mid September to mid October
Pig	mid October to mid November

ANIMALS, BIRTH HOURS, AND ELEMENTS

Rat	11 p.m. to 1 a.m.
Ox	1 a.m. to 3 a.m.
Tiger	3 a.m. to 5 a.m.
Rabbit	5 a.m. to 7 a.m.
Dragon	7 a.m. to 9 a.m.
Snake	9 a.m. to 11 a.m.
Horse	11 a.m. to 1 p.m.
Sheep	1 p.m. to 3 p.m.
Monkey	3 p.m. to 5 p.m.
Rooster	5 p.m. to 7 p.m.
Dog	7 p.m. to 9 p.m.
Pig	9 p.m. to 11 p.m.

WHAT'S THE SCORE?

Is your marriage, partnership, connection, or friendship "Made In Heaven?" Or almost as good as it gets? Or does it have just a few minor imbalances? Perhaps you have an even chance of making it together, or maybe you both need to put in a lot of work. Do you need help? If you are always at each other's throats, it feels as if it's really not working, and you want out, then just remember this:

Love can overcome anything!

You can use the little quiz given below to see how you and your lover match up under the stars. Then we'll look at what you can do about it.

Fill in the blanks, checking back with the tables on the previous pages.

YOUR ANIMALS	
Birth Year	_____
Month	_____
Hour	_____
YOUR PARTNER'S ANIMALS	
Birth Year	_____
Month	_____
Hour	_____

How do you score?

Using the following table, along with the Triangles of Friends (see fig. 5.1 on page 134) and the Circle of Rivals (see fig. 5.2 on page 135), determine your partnership score for astrological compatibility of your birth years, birth months, and birth hours.

SCORING GUIDE	
Born in the Triangle of Friends	Score 5
Neither Friends, Rivals, nor Neighbors	Score 4
Neighbors	Score 3
Share the same animal	Score 2
Born Rivals	Score 1

Year Score	_____
Month Score	_____
Hour Score	_____
Total	_____

THE MEANING OF YOUR STAR SCORE	
15	Marriage made in heaven
13–14	Almost as good as it gets
11–12	Minor imbalances
9–10	Even chances
7–8	Needs work
5–6	Get help
3	Love can overcome anything

What You Can Do about It

Even if the stars you were born under don't indicate your chances are good, all is not lost. Although you cannot change the stars, you can change yourself. In fact, you have already changed yourself. You have grown and developed since birth as you have lived your life in this world and adapted to circumstances. Utilizing the secrets of the five elements can help you smooth out the differences and give you the choice you didn't have about your birth (although some do say: "No, another time").

ELEMENTAL RELATIONSHIPS

How well do you know your lover? How do you know your lover's element? Think of the element, think of the person. Although we are each born under an element, what happens in our lives can affect it. So rather than relying on birth elements, think of what your lover is like now to see where he or she fits in the elemental pattern.

> What is fire like? What does it do? Fire warms and comforts, burns and destroys, dances like flame, cannot be grasped.
>
> Earth is serene, balanced, earthy! Living with it, we don't notice it hurtling round the sun at thousands of miles an hour.
>
> Metal is bright, hard, and sharp; it can cut and contain, reflect and inspire. And metal can be melted and shaped.
>
> Water can be still or stormy, destructive or compliant. Water fits into anything; it can turn to ice or steam, tears or tidal waves.
>
> Wood has focus and direction, competes for light, and grows in all directions.

Balance your relationship by understanding the interplay of the elements of your two natures. The mystery is solved of why one partner always seems to give—or take—more than the other. It might just be the way nature intended. But this doesn't sentence you to permanent imbalance. Your year, month, and hour of birth are in the past, fixed in the stars, but life is lived in the present.

Use awareness of the Cycle of Support between elements to guide your response to situations, to smooth out the imbalances, and harmonize your relationship (fig. 5.3). The circle moves from the top clockwise from the Firebird—fire, to the Golden Phoenix—earth, the White Tiger—metal, Black Tortoise—water, and Dragon—wood.

Cycle of Support

The sun, fire, nourishes and brings life to the earth
Deep within earth, metal is born
From the rock of metal springs water
Water feeds plant life, wood
And wood is the fuel for fire

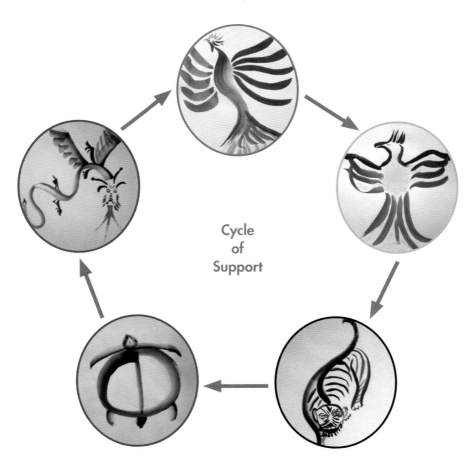

Fig. 5.3. Fire—earth—metal—water—wood

Play with the Lines of Control to soften your differences (fig. 5.4).

Lines of Control

Fire melts metal
Metal cuts wood
Wood grips earth
Earth directs water
Water regulates fire

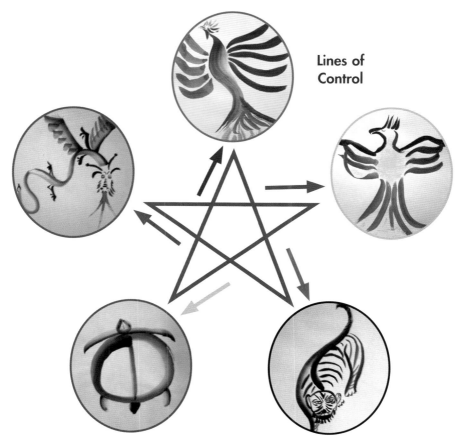

Lines of Control

Fig. 5.4. Fire—earth—metal—water—wood

What is your lover's element? Are you supporting them, or they you? You can play with support and control to restore harmony.

HOW ARE YOU WITH EACH OTHER?

Is your relationship in the Cycle of Support or governed by the Lines of Control?

If it is in the Cycle, then one of you is more the giver and the other more a receiver. If it is governed by the Lines of Control, then one controls and the other is controlled. These are natural ways of interaction and seeing the nature of your relationship can help you understand one another.

Problems come up when the receiver wants more than the giver can give, becoming a greedy child, or when the giver gives less than the receiver needs, so the receiver becomes a needy child, when the controller over-controls or the controlled one rebels.

You can help each other to work out such problems if you begin by relating the imbalances to your star-score. That will give you an idea of what to do for each other to harmonize your partnership.

If you cannot agree on each other's current predominant element, rather than birth element, just think about how you both respond to stress. If you respond as described in the left column of the following table, then the likely element is that shown in the right column.

STRESS RESPONSE	ELEMENT
Impatience, vindictiveness, hysteria	Fire
Cold detachment, weeping, silence	Metal
Anger, roughness, shouting	Wood
Worry, complaining, whining	Earth
Fear, avoidance, sighing	Water

Of course nobody is just one element. We are each made of all five but in different proportions. By identifying the predominant one you might better understand your partner's moods and your own.

HOW SEXY
IS YOUR LOVER?

What do you find sexy in your lover's face, or in any face, for that matter? What attracts you about a face? What turns you on? And what puts you off? Which of the features shown (fig. 5.5) do you find attractive? Do the ones you like have anything in common?

Do you see any resemblance between any features shown in the figure and any other parts of the body? Facial features are the "flowers

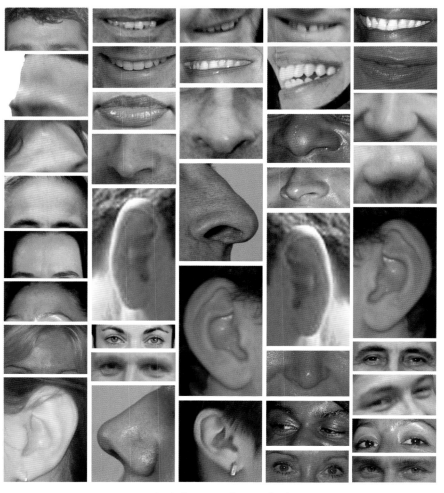

Fig. 5.5. Which features do you find attractive?

of the organs" and connect with the elements and their associated senses.

ELEMENT	SENSE	FEATURE	ORGANS
Fire	taste	tongue	heart, small intestine
Earth	touch	mouth	spleen, stomach
Metal	smell	nose	lungs, large intestine
Water	hearing	ears	kidneys, bladder
Wood	sight	eyes	liver, gallbladder

Facial features reveal the strength and weaknesses of the elements of a person's birth. Face reading is used in all branches of Chinese medicine to diagnose a person's constitutional element. In this technique, particular notice is taken of such features as a prominent philtrum or distinct earlobes (fig. 5.6).

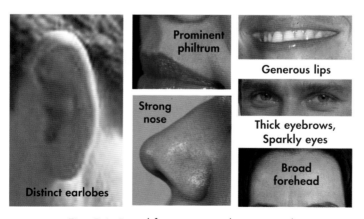

Fig. 5.6. Facial features reveal strong and weak elements of a person's birth.

You can use face reading to diagnose your lover, or even to screen potential partners! With this knowledge you can gain power: power to understand your lover and perhaps even yourself, which can guide you in adapting your lifestyle to your nature. Combined with the Taoist star chart these insights will give you the best possible chance of making the right choice.

Reading the Signs

Signs of Arousal

His

Jade Stalk grows

- Heavy
- Large
- Hard

When hot the Jade Stalk is ready to enter the Yin Gate.

Hers

- Face flushed
- Nipples hard
- Husky voice

When the Yin Gate is wet within it is ready to receive the Jade Stalk.

Theirs

- Holding breath
- Nostrils flare
- Mouth opens
- Body trembles
- Sweating
- Eyes close

They begin hugging, stretching, grasping, moaning, opening, sucking, rubbing, smiling, clutching tight.

It is easy to see the signs of arousal. But what might put you off? The senses work both ways: for example, you might be excited by the smell of sex but put off by other body odors. Senses and emotions pull

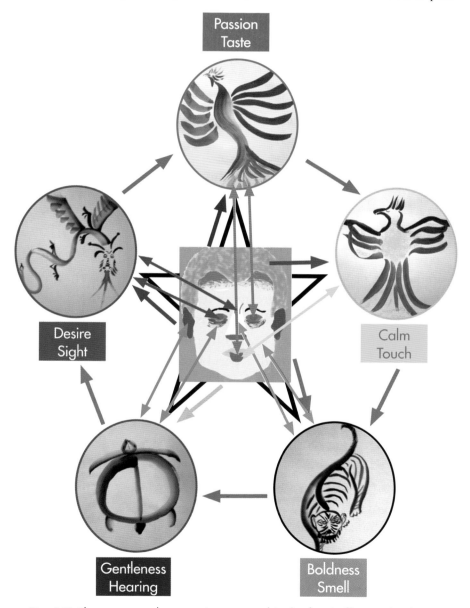

Fig. 5.7. The senses and organs (represented in the face) affect each other in the Cycle of Support and Lines of Control.

you together or push you apart: you are overwhelmed with desire, which leads you to passion, but passion is destroyed if your lover says (that is, you hear) the wrong thing at the wrong time, such as the name of an ex-lover at the moment of climax. The feelings of both you and your partner are influenced by what you see, hear, taste, smell, and touch.

You can gain great insight in how to achieve harmony by observing how the senses and organs (represented in the face) affect each other in the Cycles of Support and Lines of Control (see fig. 5.7 on page 147).

This is valuable information, which will enable you to read the signs. Now you have the knowledge to become a far more effective lover!

ENERGY VAMPIRES

Vampires are people/beings who feed off your energy. Everyone feeds off the energy of others to a greater or lesser degree because the business of life is itself a sharing. Vampires make a habit of it: they try to make all the streets one-way, toward them.

Sexual vampirism enjoyed a period of fashion in the Imperial Court of ancient China. One test of a Taoist master seeking appointment to the court was his ability to draw in the contents of a wine glass through his penis. This demonstrated his ability to leech the life force from a partner during sexual intercourse. Having shown that he had mastered the technique, he was expected to teach it to the Yellow Emperor who had at his disposal the life force of hundreds of wives and concubines.

By accumulating the chi of many others, the emperor sought to enhance his own chi and thereby attain immortality. With the same objective the Queen Mother of the West enjoyed hundreds of young men.

Both the Yellow Emperor and the Queen Mother of the West died at a ripe old age. Yes, they both died.

Sexual vampires of our times may have their own, different agenda. How can you recognize such a person? Most sexual vampires are that way unconsciously and it is not hard to recognize them by their needy, clinging, dominant, or submissive symptoms. These you can cope with in whatever way your instinct or experience tells you.

But you need to beware of the conscious vampire: one who seeks to draw your sexual essence, your life force, within and give nothing back. Here are the signs of such a person:

- A preference to make love in the sitting position, from which it is easier to practice such techniques
- As climax approaches, he will seem to emotionally withdraw into his own world. His heart will not beat faster. He will connect the energy centers and seek to hold your gaze. Looking into his eyes you will see, not the surrender of a lover, but the avarice of a feeding soul. These signs can appear in a woman as well.
- If the sexual vampire is a man, he will not ejaculate but, as his moment comes, will straighten his back. His whole body will stiffen. You may feel a sense of suction below as he holds his breath and sucks in your life force.
- If the sexual vampire is a woman, her head will not go back in ecstasy. She will draw in her chin and contain her orgasm within herself. You may feel intense suction below as she squeezes your life force out of you and into her.
- Whether male or female, neither will appear tired, weak, or drained after climax. Instead this person will have taken your juices to anoint his or her own chakra energy centers.

These, however, are the extremes. There are many loving ways of doing these practices. How do you protect yourself? Two things you must do and both are necessary: close your eyes and give, surrender into love, your own love for yourself, your lover, and all beings. Your lover's spirit will understand, as will you, that *Love Is All* and such techniques and energy-games are as nothing in the world of love.

SEX MAGIC

Sex magic offers many powerful ways to enhance a relationship but be careful not to do anything with or to another person without their consent. If sex magic is done without a person's knowledge it is unlikely to work anyway, so do not worry if you know nothing, for here ignorance is bliss. But if you wish to eat of the fruit of the Tree of Knowledge, read on, so that you may know if another is trying to perform sex magic on you.

Images, locks of hair, and clippings of nails are just as effective in potions and spells for love as they are for doing harm. Their power lies in the belief in the object.

If you want to use sex magic beneficially to support your love, then you and your partner can practice "magical ties." Of course, these often happen naturally between lovers.

Magical Ties that Bind
in the Act of Love

In the arousal phase:
Clasping each other's energy centers
Connecting your tongues
Breathing each other's breath

At the moment of climax:
Gazing into each other's left eye
Coming together
Speaking your love
Focusing on merging your spirits

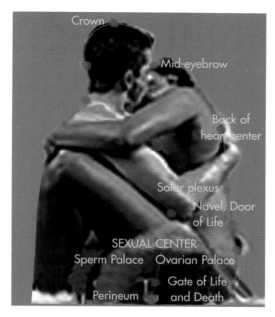

Fig. 5.8. Classical Taoist tantric position
known as Yab-Yum or Maithuna

The classical Taoist tantric position known as Yab-Yum or Maithuna facilitates these practices (fig. 5.8).

Psychic Health Warning

What Spirit Joins Together
Stays Joined Together!

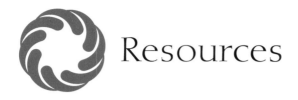

Resources

THE UNIVERSAL
TAO TRAINING CENTER

The Tao Garden Resort and Training Center in northern Thailand is the home of Master Chia and serves as the worldwide headquarters for Universal Tao activities. This integrated wellness, holistic health, and training center is situated on eighty acres surrounded by the beautiful Himalayan foothills near the historic walled city of Chiang Mai. The serene setting includes flower and herb gardens ideal for meditation, open-air pavilions for practicing Chi Kung, and a health and fitness spa.

The center offers classes year round, as well as summer and winter retreats. It can accommodate two hundred students, and group leasing can be arranged. For information worldwide on courses, books, products, and other resources, see below.

Universal Healing Tao Center

274 Moo 7, Luang Nua, Doi Saket, Chiang Mai,
    50220 Thailand

Tel: (66)(53) 495-596 Fax: (66)(53) 495-852

E-mail: universaltao@universal-tao.com

Website: www.universal-tao.com

Tao Garden Health Spa & Resort

E-mail: info@tao-garden.com,
   taogarden@hotmail.com

Website: www.tao-garden.com

ZEN SHIATSU AND HEALING TAO

London Tao Center and Zen School of Shiatsu

68 Great Eastern Street, London EC2A 3JT,
   England, United Kingdom

Tel & Fax: (44) (0) 700 078 1195

E-mail: healingtao@btinternet.com

Website: www.learn-shiatsu.co.uk

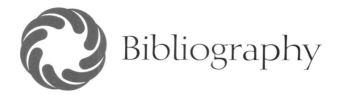 Bibliography

Allende, Isabel. *Aphrodite*. New York: HarperCollins, 1998.

Beinfield, Harriet, and Efrem Korngold. *Between Heaven & Earth*. New York: Ballantine Books, 1991.

Beresford-Cooke, Carola. *Shiatsu Theory and Practice*. London: Churchill Livingstone, 1996.

Chia, Mantak. *Chi Nei Tsang: Chi Massage for the Vital Organs*. Rochester, Vt.: Destiny Books, 2007.

———, and Maneewan Chia, Douglas Abrams, and Rachel Carlton Abrams. *MultiOrgasmic Couple*. New York: HarperCollins, 2002.

———, and William Wei. *Sexual Reflexology*. Rochester, Vt.: Destiny Books, 2003.

Douglas, Nik, and Penny Slinger. *Sexual Secrets*. Rochester, Vt.: Destiny Books, 1999.

Fall, Simon. *As Snowflakes Fall: Shiatsu as Spiritual Practice*. Devon, UK: Hazelwood Press, 1996.

Frater, U. D. *Secrets of Sex Magic*. Woodbury, Minn.: Llewellyn Publications, 1995.

Herne, Richard. *Magick, Shamanism and Taoism*. Woodbury, Minn.: Llewellyn Publications, 2001.

Hix, Sue. *Fourteen Classical Meridians*. Peterborough, UK: Rosewell Publications, 1998.

Jarrett, Lonny S. *Nourishing Destiny: The Inner Tradition of Chinese Medicine*. Stockbridge, Mass.: Spirit Path Press, 1998.

Lai, Hsi. *Sexual Teachings of the White Tigress*. Rochester, Vt.: Destiny Books, 2001.

Lau, Theodora. *Chinese Horoscopes Guide to Relationships*. New York: Doubleday, 1997.

Matsumoto, Kiiko, and Stephen Birch. *Hara Diagnosis: Reflections on the Sea.* Taos, N. Mex.: Paradigm Publications, 1988.

Wile, Douglas. *Art of the Bedchamber.* New York: State University of New York Press, 1982.

Xinnong, Cheng, ed., *Chinese Acupuncture and Moxibustion.* Beijing: Foreign Language Press, 1980.

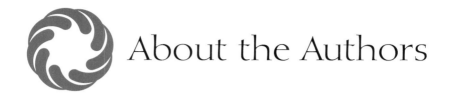 About the Authors

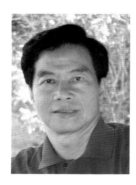

MANTAK CHIA

Mantak Chia has been studying the Taoist approach to life since childhood. His mastery of this ancient knowledge, enhanced by his study of other disciplines, has resulted in the development of the Universal Tao System, which is now being taught throughout the world.

Mantak Chia was born in Thailand to Chinese parents in 1944. When he was six years old, he learned from Buddhist monks how to sit and "still the mind." While in grammar school he learned traditional Thai boxing, and soon went on to acquire considerable skill in Aikido, Yoga, and Tai Chi. His studies of the Taoist way of life began in earnest when he was a student in Hong Kong, ultimately leading to his mastery of a wide variety of esoteric disciplines, with the guidance of several masters, including Master I Yun, Master Meugi, Master Cheng Yao Lun, and Master Pan Yu. To better understand the mechanisms behind healing energy, he also studied Western anatomy and medical sciences.

Master Chia has taught his system of healing and energizing

practices to tens of thousands of students and trained more than two thousand instructors and practitioners throughout the world. He has established centers for Taoist study and training in many countries around the globe. In June of 1990, he was honored by the International Congress of Chinese Medicine and Qi Gong (Chi Kung), which named him the Qi Gong Master of the Year.

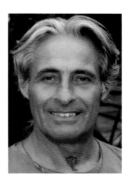

KRIS DEVA NORTH

Master of the Zen School, Kris Deva North has been involved in healing meditation since 1972 and Taoist practice since 1987. In 1993 he cofounded the Zen School of Shiatsu and London Tao Centre.

As the UK representative of the Taoist Master Mantak Chia, Kris integrates shamanic, tantric, and Taoist traditions with modern life-training techniques, from the Mind Dynamics of the 1970s to state-of-the-art neurolinguistic programming of the new millennium. His experiences range from living with Kali-worshippers of Nepal to traveling with a Thai Buddhist monk, from satsang with Shiva saddhus in the Himalayas to study with shamans of Africa, North America, and Hawaii, from study with Aboriginal men of high degree in Australia to darshan with the Dalai Lama, and from witnessing last rites in Varanasi to puja with the brahmins of Pushkar.

TV appearances include: *Bliss,* Emma Freud's series on sex and religion; Nick Hancock's *Sex and Stopping: History of Contraception;*

Carlton TV *City Survival Guide*; and Channel 4 *Extreme Celebrity Detox*.

Published articles include "Zen as a Philosophical Discipline," "Taoist Teaching, Taoist Practice, Taoist Life," "An Overview of Chi Nei Tsang," "Shiatsu—Ancient Medicine for the 21st Century," "Calabash of Light—Hawaiian Huna Healing," and the definitive interview with Mantak Chia, a modern Taoist Master. This is his first book.

www.healing-tao.co.uk
www.learn-shiatsu.co.uk

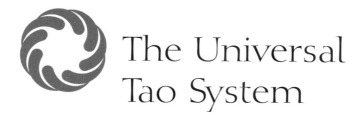

The Universal Tao System

The ultimate goal of Taoist practice is to transcend physical boundaries through the development of the soul and the spirit within the human. That is also the guiding principle behind the Universal Tao, a practical system of self-development that enables individuals to complete the harmonious evolution of their physical, mental, and spiritual bodies. Through a series of ancient Chinese meditative and internal energy exercises, the practitioner learns to increase physical energy, release tension, improve health, practice self-defense, and gain the ability to heal him- or herself and others. In the process of creating a solid foundation of health and well-being in the physical body, the practitioner also creates the basis for developing his or her spiritual potential by learning to tap into the natural energies of the sun, moon, earth, stars, and other environmental forces.

The Universal Tao practices are derived from ancient techniques rooted in the processes of nature. They have been gathered and integrated into a coherent, accessible system for well-being that works directly with the life force, or chi, that flows through the meridian system of the body.

Master Chia has spent years developing and perfecting techniques for teaching these traditional practices to students around the world through ongoing classes, workshops, private instruction, and healing sessions, as well as books and video and audio products. Further information can be obtained at **www.universal-tao.com.**

Good Chi • Good Heart • Good Intention

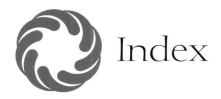 Index

Page numbers in *italics* represent illustrations.

Abdominal Breathing, 128–29, *129*
air, 11
ancestral chi, 38
arousal
    different cycles of, 9
    signs of, 146–48, *147–48*
atmospherics, 56

becoming, 11
birth time, 136–37
birth years, 132–33
Black Tortoise, 34, *34*
bladder, 11
Blue Tortoise, 34, *34*
Breast Massage, 114–15, *114–15*,
    130, *130*
Breast Palace. *See* ST 17
Bubbling Spring. *See* KD 1
Bum Squeezing, 128, *128*

Calm the Mind and Promote
    Relaxation, 84–85, *84–85*
Central Altar. *See* CV 17
Central Palace. *See* LU 1
chi, 6

Ch'in Dynasty, sexuality and, 7
Chou Dynasty, sexuality and, 7
Circle of Rivals, *135*
Classic of Internal Medicine, 5, 8
compatibility, factors effecting,
    131–32
    birth years, 132–33
    elements and, 140–42, *141–42*, 143
    friends and rivals, 134–35, *134–35*
    scoring of, 137–39
Conception Vessel, 51–53, *51–53*,
    54, *54*
Connecting Fire and Water Using
    Points GV 11 and GV 3, 62–63,
    62–63
Connecting Heaven and Earth
    Using GV 17 and GV 1, 66–67,
    66–67
Connecting the Kidney Meridian
    to the Gate of Life and Death,
    70–71, *70–71*
Connecting the Sea of Chi with the
    Sea of Tranquility, 96–97, *96–97*
Connecting the Valley of Delight
    and GV 14, 64–65, *64–65*

Connecting the Yin Tang and the Jade Pillow, 98–99, *98–99*

Connecting Your Lover's Bubbling Spring to Your Heart Fire, 89–91, *89–91*

Connecting Your Lover's Door of Life and Spirit's Palace Gate, 82–83, *82–83*

Connect to Your Lover's Sexual Essence, 76–77, *76–77*

CV 1, 26, 53, *53*, 70–71, *70–71*, 82–83, *82–83*, 88, 111, *111*

CV 2, 52, 111, *111*

CV 3, 110, *110*

CV 6, 52–53, *52–53*, 96–97, *96–97*, 109, *109*

CV 8, 52

CV 14, 52, 89–90, *89–90*

CV 17, 52, 86–87, *86–87*, 96–97, *96–97*

Cycle of Support, 13–15, *13–14*, *141*, 148

Cyclic Gate. *See* LV 14

Decision Maker. *See* Gall Bladder meridian

Door of Life, 47. *See also* GV 4

Dragon, 40–41, *40*

Dynasties, sexuality and, 7–8

earth element, 5, 11, 24

meridians of, 24–28, *24–28*

Eighth Flower, 111, *111*

elements. *See also* five elements

elements, birth time and, 136–37

energy channels, 2–3, *3*

energy vampires, 148–50

eyes, 16

face, massage of, 100–101, *100–101*

facial features, 144–45, *147*

fall, 11

fear, 34

Fifth Flower, 108, *108*

fire, 5, 11, 15–23

Firebird, 15–16, *16*

fire element, meridians of, 16–23, *16–23*

First Flower, 104, *104*

five elements, 5, 11

birth time and, 136–37

emotions and, 13–15, *13–15*

meridians and, 12–13, *12*

relationships and, 143

five phases of energy, 11, *11*

foot-belly massage, 92–93, *92–93*

Fourth Flower, 107, *107*

friends and rivals, 134–35, *134–35*

Full-body Shiatsu Love Massage

Moving Down the Back (part 1), 61–77, *61–77*

Moving Down to Heaven (part 5), 103–11, *103–11*

Moving Up the Left Side (part 4), 102, *102*

Moving Up the Right Side (part 2), 78–85, *78–85*

gallbladder, 11

Gall Bladder meridian, 44–46, *44–46*

Gate of Life and Death. *See* CV 1

GB 21, 45–46, *45–46*

GB 24, 45–46, *45–46*, 92–93, *93*, 106, *106*

GB 30, 45–46, *45–46*, 72–73, 80–81, *80–81*

Generate Desire, 78–79, *78–79*

Golden Phoenix, 24, *24*

Governing Vessel, 47–50, *47–50*, 54

Great Palace. *See* CV 14

Great Rushing. *See* LV 3

Great Stream. *See* KD 3

guardian animals, *141–42*

    Black Tortoise, 34, *34*

    Dragon, 40–41, *40*

    Firebird, 15–16, *16*

    Golden Phoenix, 24, *24*

    White Tiger, *29*

GV 1, 48, *48*, 50, *50*, 66–67, *66–67*

GV 2, 48, *48*, 50, *50*, 64–65, *64–65*, 82–83, *82–83*

GV 3, 48, *48*, 50, *50*, 62–63, *63*

GV 4, 48–49, *48–49*

GV 11, 48–49, *48–49*, 62–63, *63*

GV 14, 48–49, *48–49*, 64–65, *64–65*

GV 15, 48–49, *48–49*, 84–85, *84–85*, 86, *86*

GV 17, 48, *48*, 66–67, *66–67*, 98–99, *98–99*

harvesting, 11

heart, 11

Heart meridian, 16–17, *16–17*

Heart Protector meridian, 22–23, *22–23*

Heavenly Axis. *See* ST 25

HP 8, 23, *23*, 68–69, *68–69*, 74–75, *74–75*, 84–85, *84–85*, 86–87, *86–87*, 98, *98*

Huang Ti (Yellow Emperor), 4–5, *4*

immortality, sexuality and, 6

Indian summer, 11

Inner Alchemy, 7

Internal Egg exercise, 117–24, *117–23*

internal organs, 11

jade eggs, 117–18

Jade Pillow. *See* GV 17

Jade Stalk, 41

Joining Two Fire Meridians, 68–69, *68–69*

Jumping Circle. *See* GB 30

KD 1, 38–39, *39*, 76–77, *76–77*, 89–91, *89–91*, 92

KD 3, 38–39, *39*, 76–77, *76–77*

KD 11, 38–39, *39*, 94–95, *94–95*

Kidney meridian, 38–39, *38–39*

kidneys, 11

Kunlun Mountain. *See* UB 60

Labor's Love. *See* HP 8

large intestine, 11

Large Intestine meridian, 32–33, *32–33*

Lasting Strength. *See* GV 1

Later Han Dynasty, sexuality and, 7

LI 4, 32–33, *33*

life force. *See* chi

Lines of Control, 13–15, *13–14*, 142, 148
liver, 11
Liver meridian, 41–43, *41–43*
lover, preparing, 56–58, *56–58*
Love-Shiatsu, 4
numerology of, 59–61, *59–61*
preparations for, 55–58, *56–58*
LU 1, 30–31, *31*
lubricant, 55
Lung meridian, 30–31, *30–31*
lungs, 11
LV 3, 42–43, *42–43*, 90
LV 4, 42–43, *42–43*, 90
LV 8, 42–43, *42–43*, 88, *88*
LV 9, 42–43, *42–43*, 78–79, *78–79*
LV 12, 42–43, *42–43*, 94–95, *94–95*
LV 14, 42–43, *42–43*, 92–93, *93*, 105, *105*

massage. *See* Full-body Shiatsu Love Massage
Massage of the Dragon Pearls, 125–26, *125–26*
Massage of the Nine Flowers, 26
Massaging the Perineum, 129–30, *129–30*
Master of the Heart. *See* Heart Protector meridian
mead, 56
meridians, 6, 12–13, *12*
metal element, 5, 11, 29–33
meridians of, 30–33, *30–33*
Microcosmic Orbit, 48
Middle Barrier. *See* LV 4
Ming Men. *See* GV 4

Minister of Fun. *See* Heart Protector meridian
Moving Down the Back, 61–77, *61–77*
Moving Up the Left Side, 102, *102*

Neijing, 5, 8
Nine Flowers Massage, 52, 103–11
Ninth Flower, 111, *111*
Northern Wei, 7–8

ovaries, 116, *116*

PC muscle, 42
perineum, 129–30
perishing, 11
pregnancy, 45

Queen Mother, 6

relationships. *See* compatability, factors effecting
ripening, 11

Sea of Chi. *See* CV 6
Sea of Tranquility. *See* CV 17
seasons, 11, *11*
Second Flower, 105
Secret Instructions of the Jade Bedchamber, 8
Self-Shiatsu, 112–13, *112–13*
for everyone, 128–30, *128–30*
for men, 124–27, *124–27*
for women, 114–24, *115–23*
Send Waves of Bliss through Your Lover, 86–87, *86–87*

senses, *2*

Seventh Flower, 110, *110*

sex and sexuality

immortality and, 6

as servant, 7

sexiness, 144–48

sex magic, 150–51

shiatsu. *See* Full-body Shiatsu
Love Massage; Self-Shiatsu

Shoulder Well. *See* GB 21

SI 11, 68–69, *68–69*

sight, 40–41

Sixth Flower, 109, *109*

small intestine, 11

Small Intestine meridian, 18–19,
18–19

SP 6, 28, *28*, 78–79, *78–79*

SP 9, 28, *28*

SP 12, 28, *28*, 94–95, *94–95*

Spiral Massage of the Buttocks,
72–73, *72–73*

Spirit's Palace Gate. *See* CV 8

spleen, 11

Spleen meridian, 27–28, *27–28*

spring, 11

ST 17, 25–26, *25–26*, 102, *102*,
104, *104*

ST 21, 26, *26*, 92–93, *93*, 107,
107

ST 25, 26, *26*, 92–93, *93*, 108,
108

stomach, 11

Stomach meridian, 24–26, *24–26*

stone eggs, 117–18

stress, 8–9

Stretching the Stalk, 126–27, *127*

Stroking the Flowers of the
Elemental Organs in the Face,
100–101, *100–101*

Sui Dynasty, 8

summer, 11

Supporting Palace. *See* UB 36

Tang Dynasty, 8

Tao and Taoism, 7–8

Taoist sexual practices, origins of,
4–8

Tapping the Pearls, 127

TH 1, 21, *21*

Third Flower, 106, *106*

Three Kingdoms and Six
Dynasties, 7

tongue, 16

Triangle of Friends, *134*

Triple Heater meridian, 20–21,
20–21

UB 23, 36, *36*, 70–71, *70–71*

UB 32, 36–37, *36–37*

UB 36, 36–37, *36–37*, 80–81, *80–81*

UB 37, 36–37, *36–37*, 74–75, *74–75*

UB 60, 36–37, *36–37*, 76–77, *76–77*

Urinary Bladder meridian, 35–37,
35–37

uterus, 116, *116*

Valley of Delight. *See* GV 2

Warming up the Jade Stalk, 125,
125

Warming Your Lover's Urinary
Bladder Meridian, 80–81, *80–81*

water element, 5, 11, 34
  meridians of, 35–39, *35–39*
White Tiger, 29, *29*
winter, 11
women, Self-Shiatsu for, 114–24,
  115–23
wood element, 5, 11, 40–41

Yab-Yum, 151, *151*
yang meridians
  Gall Bladder, 44–46, *44–46*
  Governing Vessel, 47–50, *47–50*
  Large Intestine, 32–33, *32–33*
  Small Intestine, 18–19, *18–19*
  Stomach, 24–26, *24–26*

Triple Heater, 20–21, *20–21*
  Urinary Bladder, 35–37, *35–37*
Yellow Emperor, 4–5, *4*, 6
yin and yang, 5, 8, 12–13
Yin Gate, 41
yin meridians
  Conception Vessel, 51–53,
    51–53
  Heart, 16–17, *16–17*
  Heart Protector, 22–23, *22–23*
  Kidney, 38–39, *38–39*
  Liver, 41–43, *41–43*
  Lung, 30–31, *30–31*
  Spleen, 27–28, *27–28*
Yin Tang, 98–99, *98–99*

BOOKS OF RELATED INTEREST

Sexual Reflexology
Activating the Taoist Points of Love
by Mantak Chia and WillIam U. Wei

Healing Love through the Tao
Cultivating Female Sexual Energy
by Mantak Chia

Chi Kung for Prostate Health and Sexual Vigor
A Handbook of Simple Exercises and Techniques
by Mantak Chia and William U. Wei

Chi Kung for Women's Health and Sexual Vitality
A Handbook of Simple Exercises and Techniques
by Mantak Chia and William U. Wei

Karsai Nei Tsang
Therapeutic Massage for the Sexual Organs
by Mantak Chia

The Alchemy of Sexual Energy
Connecting to the Universe from Within
by Mantak Chia

Tantric Sex for Men
Making Love a Meditation
by Diana Richardson and Michael Richardson

Tantric Orgasm for Women
by Diana Richardson

Inner Traditions • Bear & Company
P.O. Box 388
Rochester, VT 05767
1-800-246-8648
www.InnerTraditions.com

Or contact your local bookseller